The Ghoraa and Limbic Exercise

Principles and practice of limbic exercise based on intuitive insights of the ancients and an understanding of the energy dynamics of fat-burning and sugar-burning exercises, health and disease

How to do slow and sustained exercise and eat life span foods to lose weight and enjoy greater energy, better health and longer life

Majid Ali, M.D.

Associate Professor of Pathology (Adj)
College of Physicians and Surgeons of Columbia University, New York
Director, Department of Pathology, Immunology and Laboratories
Holy Name Hospital, Teaneck, New Jersey
Consulting Physician
Institute of Preventive Medicine, Denville, New Jersey
Fellow, Royal College of Surgeons of England
Diplomate, American Board of Environmental Medicine
Diplomate, American Board of Chelation Therapy

Library of Congress Cataloging-in-Publication Data

Ali, Majid
The Ghoraa and Limbic Exercise Majid Ali.--1st ed.

Includes bibliographical references and index
1. Limbic (Fat-Burning) Exercises
2. Cortical (Sugar-Burning) Exercises
3. Up-Regulation of Fat-Burning Enzymes
4. Limbic Lengthening of Connective Tissue
5. Limbic Pacing
6. Limbic Exercise for Chronic Fatigue, Heart Disease,
Arthritis and Other Disorders

ISBN 1-879131-02-1
10 9 8 7 6 5 4 3 2 1

Published in the USA by

IPM PRESS
95 East Main Street, Denville, N.J. 07843
(201) 586-9191

I devote this book to the gentle guiding energy of the *presence* that always surrounds each one of us.

The longer Levin mowed, the oftener he experienced those moments of oblivion when it was not his arms which swung the scythe but the scythe seemed to mow of itself, a body full of life and consciousness of its own, and as though by magic, without a thought being given to it, the work did itself regularly and carefully. These were the most blessed moments.

Leo Tolstoy in *Anna Karenina*

CONTENTS

Preface

Mankind needs the language of silence today more than at any time during its history; likewise, we need optimal regulation of life span enzymes more than ever. As I delved deeper into those two areas, I recognized that one cannot be achieved without the other. I describe in this book how the idea of combining the language of silence with slow, sustained exercise was a gift to me from a ghoraa, a horse that pulls a tonga — a poor man's buggy — in Pakistan. I used to ride tongas whenever I visited my family in Kirto, my village in Pakistan.

The central issue in physical fitness today is not that we do not fully understand the health benefits of exercise. This book is not intended merely to detail them for those few who may still not know them. The main issue in fitness today is that most people are unable to exercise regularly. If inertia and boredom or lack of energy and poor tissue conditioning are the reasons, how can those problems be resolved so that exercise may be made a part of our day? This book is intended to provide answers to these questions and offer some guidance.

How Does an African Message Carrier Run?

In what state of energy is he in? How does an American executive run? What does his cluttered mind demand from his tired and hurt tissues? The African runs for miles and miles without perspiration, hyperventilation and heart palpitations. He runs with cadence, without tearing his ligaments and without rupturing his muscles. The American runs with a heavy burden of goals, and often returns with sore legs, sprained ankles and bruised ego. Can the American run like the African? If not, why not?

The African messenger runs for miles in the bush under a blazing sun. He moves in a rhythm, his stick in delicate balance with his frame. He is a part of the wilderness around him. He is in communion with some larger *presence* around him. He may not put it in words that we can understand, but he *knows* something about this *presence*. At the end of the run, he neither hyperventilates nor perspires. There is serenity on his face. The American executive runs to the bidding of his cardiologist. He runs to attain 70% of his maximal aerobic capacity or some other similarly frivolous number. He has been admonished that anything less than that will not work. He lumbers along the sidewalk, breathing the exhaust of cars rushing past him. His face is contorted, his legs tremble, his feet scream with discomfort. But the gladiator goes on, on and on, in pursuit of his percentage points. He runs as if he is running for his life. Little does he realize that he *does* run for his life.

A Physician Runs for Cholesterol

A physician colleague had a blood cholesterol level test done as a part of a routine physical examination. His cholesterol level turned out to be 265 mg/dl. His cardiologist expressed concern about this value, and firmly advised him to embark upon a program of daily exercise for at least 20 minutes. Without exercise, the cardiologist told my colleague, he would need one of the cholesterol-lowering drugs. As he talked about his ambitious exercise program, I wondered how much exercise he needed to achieve this goal. He was in his mid-forties. If he was going to live to be ninety, I computed in my mind, he needed to do exercise on 16,425 different occasions. How does anyone go about devoting 16,425 periods of exercise to keep his cholesterol level low? I wondered. What were his chances of succeeding at that?

A *minute* is not a small period of time when one *has* to do what he would rather not do. I know how quickly the patterns of energy of the heart, muscle, skin and other body organs change with minimal stresses. I explain such changes in the electromagnetic patterns to all my patients in my auto-regulation laboratory. These events require thousands of adrenaline and related neurotransmitter molecules. It is worth noting that 16,425 periods of exercise of 20 minutes each come to 328,500 minutes of exercise. How many billions of stress molecules are we talking about? Or is it trillions?

Over 300,000 minutes of unwanted exercise! That is an awfully long time for the arteries to be violated by the mind as it computes and recomputes the desired changes in the blood cholesterol levels. I wondered what possible life span benefits would accrue were my colleague to succeed in lowering this level — especially when it is not at all clear to me (and my colleagues in nutritional medicine) what the real danger of heart attack is when the blood cholesterol level is 265. I wondered how much he would tighten his arteries worrying about his cholesterol level. I wondered how his tightened arteries would suffocate his tissues. I felt a surge of pity.

Then I realized that his body tissues were not going to be punished to any serious degree. No one can go through years of such frivolous notions without finally recognizing the utter stupidity of it all. Tissues simply do not allow the mind to molest them for long. I felt reassured. Biology is not subservient to the contortions of the mind. No one can endure the punishment of such exercise programs for decades just to lower his cholesterol number. The tissues simply do not stand for it. Exercise is essential for optimal function of life span enzymes, but for it to be a part of one's day, it must be needed at a deeper, intuitive-visceral level. Exercise must be *giving* at every moment if it is to be done regularly. It is simply not possible to exercise every day, every week, every month, every year, for forty or fifty years, to lower cholesterol level, and possibly prolong life by a few weeks and months.

What Is the Only Part of the Human Condition That Lies?

One simple observation has guided me in my work with limbic exercise. Tissues do not lie. I have never seen a heart that malingers or a muscle that misleads or a skin that schemes. I concluded, therefore, that distortions come from none other than the thinking mind. If the mind is the only part of the human condition that lies, I then asked myself, why should I listen to it in matters of exercise and autoregulation? This simple notion appeared to provide a reasonable framework for my work.

When man learned to observe, he learned to self-regulate. Self-regulation took different forms in different eras and in different cultures. The central observation behind it remained the same; namely, that body tissues respond when we learn to listen to them. It seemed only natural that this simple observation would be relevant to the field of physical fitness. In *The Cortical Monkey and Healing,* I describe my entry into the domain of self-regulation. Unaware of the richness of the ancient writings that chronicle man's search for truth — and inevitably of his forays into the realms of consciousness — I saw my own observations of evident value to the practice of the healing arts. The physical responses I observed clearly had a definable electrophysiologic basis.

What Is Preventive Medicine?

The thrust of this book — and of its companion volumes *The Cortical Monkey and Healing, The Butterfly and Life Span Nutrition* and *The Canary and Chronic Fatigue* — is to define some new dimensions in preventive medicine.

Few things are as discouraging as the attitude of the practitioners of drug medicine toward preventive medicine. Among themselves, they do not believe preventive medicine has any real role in their professional work. Yes, they do advise their patients to reduce stress by "relaxing", instruct them to quit smoking, drink less and lose weight if obesity exists. Some very enlightened practitioners of drug medicine even tell their patients to take a multivitamin tablet daily to prevent deficiency diseases. This is where it all ends. These practitioners of drug medicine know that none of this ever works. Hence, their belief that preventive medicine does not work.

I define preventive medicine first as a reversal of chronic health disorders with nondrug therapies, and then as health promotion. Nondrug therapies must be practiced according to the principles and practice of molecular medicine — a medicine that integrates the practice of nutritional medicine, environmental medicine, and the medicine of self-regulation and physical fitness. When this goal is achieved, then, and only then, is a patient ready to receive from his physician guidance for prevention of disease with nondrug treatment protocols. The problem is that the practitioners of drug medicine consider the practice of molecular medicine quackery, and the reversal of disease obtained with its treatment protocols as treatment of diseases that really do not exist. This is a hard criticism of my profession, but it is well-deserved.

"Thought Provoking"

The staff at IPM Press asked a colleague if he would read some parts of this manuscript and consider writing a sentence or two for promotional use. He called me and spoke many kind words about this book. His written comment that arrived a few days later included the phrase "thought provoking." The cortical monkey doesn't let up, does it? I wondered about his words. This whole book is about breaking through the stronghold of the thinking mind. It is about uncluttering the cluttered mind. "Thought provoking!" That was the furthest thing from my mind during the period of writing this book. When my associate pathologist Verna Atkins, M.D.,

___

heard about this, she mused, "Sometimes things are so off-base, that they help crystalize what the base is."

We cannot "clever-think" our way out of all our problems. There are times we need the limbic language of silence. This book is about how slow, sustained exercise can be combined with the language of silence to achieve higher physical and spiritual states.

Majid Ali, M.D.
Blairstown, New Jersey
April 5, 1993

No matter what you hear, from whom, seeking the truth in what you hear is your wisdom.

Ancient Sanskrit Writings

Chapter 1

> ## *The Cortical Monkey*
> ## *and*
> ## *The Limbic Dog*

Autoregulation, the Cortical Monkey and the Limbic Dog

The terms autoregulation, the cortical monkey and limbic dog appear throughout this book. Following are some excerpts from my previous books, *The Cortical Monkey and Healing* and *The Limbic Dog and Directed Pulses,* that will serve as a reference for these terms.

The Cortical Monkey

There is a particular species of monkey native to Karnal, my birthplace. During my childhood, these monkeys lived in our town by the hundreds. They were a nuisance for the grown-ups, but for us children they were a lot of fun. I remember my father telling me how these monkeys had a peculiar habit. They did not let their wounds heal. If one of them ever lacerated his skin, he would pick at his wound continuously. He would peel off whatever little scab did form. These wounds festered for long periods of time.

Putting Something Between the Monkey and His Wound

It has occurred to me that the first man to invent a

bandage probably got his idea from watching a monkey (or some other animal) constantly pick at his wound. It might have occurred to him that the way to let the wound heal would be to put something between the monkey and his wound. When he got hurt himself, the lesson learned from the monkey might have taken a practical turn. A bunch of leaves, perhaps of some herbal plant, might have served this purpose. This, or something similar, is likely to have been the forerunner of our modern Band-Aid.

There is something relevant in the story of Karnal monkeys to our ideas of self-regulation and healing. Time and again, I see patients who understand how their *cortical condition* throws roadblocks in the way of *limbic healing*. In our autoregulation laboratory, I demonstrate to them how their biologic profiles are composed of a host of electromagnetic or molecular events. I show them how their whole biology is sustained in an even state when they go *limbic*, and how it is thrown into turbulence when they go *cortical*. I explain to them the impact on their internal organs of *talking for control* and *listening for healing*. At intellectual and analytical levels, they seem to understand these phenomena. Yet, left to their own devices, they slide back into the calculating and competitive *cortical state*. They are unable to keep their analytical mind ("the cortical monkey") out of the way of the healing *limbic state*.

Indeed, patient and persistent work is required to break long-established cortical habits and put the cortical monkey to sleep.

Thinking Is an Intellectual Function;
Healing Is Not

In autoregulation, I do not ask my patients to think positively. In autoregulation, I strive to teach them how **not** to think. Thinking about how not to think is a catch 22. The harder we try not to think, the deeper we slide into thinking. This is where the concept of energy in autoregulation comes into play.

The theory of the value of positive thinking is well understood by most people. The obvious benefits of positive thinking notwithstanding, such thoughts by themselves, in my experience, are rarely sufficient to allow most people to reverse chronic disorders and regain health. Indeed, patients debilitated by chronic diseases and exhausted by unrelenting suffering often find the advice of positive thinking as salt on their wounds. For these reasons I do not make a practice of recommending positive thinking to very ill patients.

The concept of physical healing energy in autoregulation is often misunderstood in a society that is oriented to the chemical resolution of all health problems. Many of my patients equate the principles and practice of autoregulation to some variant of Eastern philosophy or mysticism. Fortunately, most people are able to perceive the healing energy of autoregulation in some fashion during the very first training session in my laboratory. This initial experience helps them dissipate any misgivings they might have about the true nature of the healing process involved in autoregulation. From then on, it is simply a matter of increasing the intensity of such energy and enhancing its clinical benefits.

Injured Molecules and Cells Heal with Energy; Autoregulation Is About This Energy.

The critical issue is how to become aware of this energy, how to increase its intensity and, finally, how to use it to regulate one's biology and allow the injured molecules and cells to heal. In the initial stages, it is necessary to understand clearly *what autoregulation is and what it is not.*

* *Autoregulation is healing by listening to tissues and perceiving their energy.*

* *Autoregulation is not healing by talking to tissues and thinking positively.*

The principles of self-regulation are valid for all patients and all diseases. The applications of such principles, however, require careful evaluation of the nature and extent of each patient's disease (that is, the weight and duration of the specific burdens on his biology). Different diseases cause different levels of suffering and require different degrees of effort with different time frames.

In my early clinical work with environmental medicine, I saw patients who responded poorly or not at all to the standard drug therapies. Many of them were actually made worse by drugs. Understandably, those patients were highly stressed. I set out to relieve some of their suffering by what I then thought was going to be termed "stress management." I started teaching them how to slow their hearts, open their arteries and dissolve their muscle tension. In medical terminology, such activities are referred to as autonomic functions. It seemed logical to use the term autonomic regulation for it. My patients abbreviated this to autoregulation and eventually to "autoreg."

I soon realized my patients both needed and wanted me to teach them methods for self-regulation and healing. I also recognized that self-regulation goes far beyond any ideas of autonomic regulation. I started a search for a simple term that, in practical terms, would declare my purpose.

Again, my patients solved my problem. They stayed with the term autoregulation as I experimented with different words. In the end I decided to follow their lead. Looking back, my work with autoregulation evolved in the following sequence:

1. *Stress management*
2. *Autonomic regulation*
3. *Self-regulation and healing*
4. *States of consciousness*

One of the essential lessons my patients taught me is

this: Slowing the heart rate, keeping the arteries open and slow, even breathing profoundly affect our state of mind. These basic methods of autoregulation are very effective in dissipating anger and anxiety even when that is not our intended purpose. But that is just a beginning. Autoregulation reveals the path of self-regulation and healing. A passage through the realms of self-regulation inevitably ushers a person to higher states of awareness and consciousness.

Autoregulation
Is Self-Regulation and Healing with Energy

Autoregulation is self-regulation and healing with energy — energy derived from tissues, cells and molecules. It is self-regulation with full benefits of the science and technology of modern medicine. It is self-regulation with changes that can be measured with electromagnetic, molecular and cellular techniques. When an individual practices self-regulation, *he* becomes the true judge of its efficacy, not some pseudoscientist with silly notions of double-blind cross-over methods of medical research.

Autoregulation Is Not Healing with Hypnosis, Psychoanalysis, Psychotherapy, Regression, Progression or Biofeedback

Hypnosis is a valuable treatment option. Unlike drugs,

hypnosis has never had a toxic effect on anyone. At once, the hypnotist puts the patient into a trance and puts him out of his misery. The patient obtains immediate relief, though he has no understanding of how he obtained it. It is my personal observation that the good effects of hypnosis almost always wear out with time. Continued hypnosis fails to sustain the initial benefits.

Autoregulation, by contrast, is a slow process. It generally does not offer immediate relief. Most people learn autoregulation methods over days and weeks. *However, once learned, the methods of autoregulation never lose their clinical efficacy.* Indeed, the longer a person practices autoregulation, the more profound its benefits. No one ever unlearns autoregulation. Autoregulation works even when an individual is in the throes of an acute life-threatening illness, though the benefits may be rather limited under such circumstances.

The critical difference between autoregulation and hypnosis is this: Autoregulation is a path of independence. Hypnosis and the placebo effect are the paths of dependence.

THE CORTICAL AND LIMBIC STATES

In my working model of self-regulation (and healing) in clinical medicine, I use the term "cortical state" to refer to a state of the human condition that calculates, computes, competes, cautions, creates stress, causes immune dysfunctions, and culminates in disease. I use the term "limbic state" to refer to a state of the human condition that cares and comforts, creates images of health, and allows the injured molecules, cells and tissues to heal by their own innate healing abilities.

In order to unleash the *limbic condition*'s ability to heal, it must first be freed from the relentless censor of the *cortical mind*. Switching off the thinking cortical mode is simple to understand at an intellectual level, but it requires considerable practical experience. The harder one tries not to think, the more difficult it becomes. Only very intuitive people turn out to experience exceptions to this.

An Energy-Over-Mind Approach to Healing

We often hear about the concept of healing with a mind-over-body approach. In my own work with self-regulation, I do not find this to be sufficient for reversing chronic indolent diseases. Instead, I see superior clinical results when my patients adopt an "energy-over-mind" approach, i.e., when they learn how to listen and attend to their tissues and shut out their thinking minds.

We take pride in our minds, but healing is not an intellectual function. Healing cannot be forced upon injured cells and tissues by a demanding mind. Rather, healing occurs when the tissues are set free from the ceaseless censor of the mind. My patients were unable to control their asthma and migraine attacks, lower their raised blood pressure, or reverse other chronic illnesses with a mind-over-body approach.

The Limbic Dog

A boy brought home two newborn puppies, one was white and the other gray. He fell in love with the white puppy. He put the gray puppy in a crib and held the white puppy in his hands. The white puppy kept his eyes closed. His skin was soft and his hair snow-white and delicate. The boy petted his white puppy until late evening hours. Then he asked his mother if he could put his puppy to sleep in his own bed. His mother smiled and told him that was very dangerous. The puppy could be smothered by him in his sleep. The boy understood that and gently put the puppy in his crib.

When he woke up the next morning, his puppies were awake and seemed hungry. He took the puppies out of their crib and asked his mother to teach him how to prepare their formula. As he fed them, he had eyes only for the white puppy. Then he put the puppies back into the crib, instructed his mother about their care and left for school. At school, he was distracted all day by thoughts of his white puppy. The gray puppy was not a part of his day. When the school bell rang for the last time, he ran to his home to be with his white puppy. Once home, he threw his satchel on a chair and rushed to the crib. The noise woke the puppies up. He lifted both puppies out of the crib and put them on the floor. Again, he had eyes only for the white puppy. He petted him and held him in his lap. The gray puppy moved around, unaware and unaffected by the boy's preoccupation with the white puppy. Late that night, he fed the puppies again, his eyes remaining fixed on the white puppy.

The next day was no different. The boy woke up and hurried to the crib. The puppies were sleeping. He gently petted the white puppy as it slept. Then he brought the puppies their meal. He watched every little movement the white puppy made with intent eyes. This day at school was like the previous day. He stayed deep in thoughts of his tiny white puppy. Again, the grey puppy was out of his mind. That afternoon and evening, he again played with the white puppy. The gray puppy wandered around, oblivious of the boy's preoccupation with the white puppy.

Days passed and then weeks. The boy's fondness for the white puppy seemed to grow with each passing day. The puppies grew up fast and became strong. The boy started housebreaking his puppies. That is when the boy's parents noticed that the gray puppy began to misbehave. Sometimes he looked at the boy with silent, plaintive eyes, at other times he barked without any reason. On occasion, he appeared to want to break things. On some afternoons, the gray puppy seemed to purposely throw up his food on the kitchen floor and soil the rug in the living room. That annoyed the boy's parents and they scolded him. As for the boy, he was too absorbed playing with his white puppy to want to do much with the gray puppy. Each time the gray puppy did something the boy didn't like, it further drove the boy closer to his white puppy. The more the gray puppy was scolded, the more accident-prone he became.

Months passed. The puppies grew up into little dogs. The boy's love for his white dog became deeper with each passing month. The white dog knew this. He waited for the boy to return from school all day. The afternoons were pure bliss for both of them. They played together, ate their meals together, and then went out to a nearby field for more play. The gray dog seemed to sense the closeness between the two and often became sad. Sometimes he felt angry and hurt. On most days, he kept all that to himself, but sometimes it was too much for him. It was then that there were accidents that made the boy yell at him. Some more months passed.

Then the gray dog changed. He was not sad anymore. Nor was he ever angry. No one noticed that the gray dog stopped having any accidents. He neither made a mess in the kitchen nor did he soil the rugs anymore. When the boy returned home, the gray dog stood back, watching the white dog leap to meet his little master. Sometimes when the boy's eyes fell upon the gray dog, the dog gently cocked his head or wagged his tail. That was all. The boy didn't follow it with any words. The gray dog didn't ask for anything more.

Years passed. The boy grew up into a young man and the dogs into two strong dogs. Every day, when the young man returned from work, the white dog greeted him with great excitement and leaped all over him. The gray dog stood behind, silently watching the two friends. After some time, the man went to his kitchen and cooked his meal as the white dog hovered around him. The gray dog stood still in the corner. His face bore a calm, unexpressive expression. After the meal was ready, the man ate it with his white dog and then left his house for a walk with his white dog. It was then that the gray dog walked over to the table and ate what was left behind. Then he walked out briskly to catch up with the man and his white dog. There he stood by the edge of the field, impassively looking at the man and the white dog. When it turned dark, the man and his white dog returned home, the gray dog walking several paces behind them. That was the way weeks followed the days and months followed the weeks.

One rainy day the man was driving to work when his car slid and crashed into another car. He sustained a head injury and concussion and fractured several of his ribs. Some days later, he opened his eyes and saw some fuzzy figures in white robes milling around his bed. He tried to sit up but collapsed with pangs of pain in different parts of his body. Moments later he opened his eyes and looked around the room. He saw tubes and wires running into his body parts from bottles hanging from poles and video screens on the walls. Is it a nightmare? Am I dying? he wondered. Then he saw some nurses walk by. He realized he was in a hospital. He thought back and recalled the fleeting moment of terror before his car crashed. His body shook with fear. He tried to get up, felt a sharp pain in his chest and collapsed onto his bed. Am I going to live? he asked himself as he came around the second time. He looked out of the window. The sunset filtered weakly through the mist of a late winter afternoon.

The man closed his eyes. A faint shadow of a dog appeared in the distant mist. Then the shadow sharpened into the face of a white dog. The dog looked at him with gleaming eyes. My dog, he murmured softly and opened his eyes. His face softened into a smile. A nurse passed by. Again he closed his eyes to recapture the image of his white dog and savor the moment. The dog's head reappeared. His chest heaved as he looked longingly at his dog. Love filled his whole body and everything that surrounded him. He opened his eyes and looked around. He felt calm as he looked at the pale yellow solution dripping slowly into the little chamber below the IV bottle and the blips and waves moving across the heart monitor.

The man studied the ICU room for a while and then closed his eyes again, wondering if his white-faced visitor still hung around in the mist outside his window. As his eyes closed, the image of his white dog reappeared, and then it changed. The white face of the dog became pale and then beige. Slowly the color deepened and turned darker. Suddenly there stood before him his gray dog, silent and sullen and sad. Something stirred in him. He opened his eyes in pain. The image of the head of his gray dog vanished. He looked at the faint pale sun disk through the mist and felt sadness surging within him. Slowly he closed his eyes. A sharp image hit his eyes this time. It was the picture of his puppies the day he first brought them home. Something stirred in him again, much more intensely than before. He opened his eyes but this time it was different. The image of the gray dog persisted in the mist. The gray dog peered at him with his large, soft brown eyes. Oh, my God! The words froze in his throat. How could I? How could anyone? He cried out in pain. How could anyone be so cruel? How could I have been so cruel, and for so long? He closed his eyes in deep anguish. The image of the gray dog persisted before his closed eyes. The dog looked at him with vacant eyes. The man's arms rose to reach the gray dog in the mist. The dog's image receded further back into the mist. And then the dog's eyes turned wet and there was a flood of tears in his large, brown eyes. Oh, my God! the man winced with intense pain. How could I? How could anyone? How could I? he repeated his words. But the images rolled on and on, like a homemade video. Images of a tiny gray puppy, searching for something in the eyes of a little boy. Images of a gray puppy awkwardly throwing himself at a little boy as the boy shrank back to pick up a white puppy.

Images of a puppy vomiting on a kitchen floor and urinating on a rug. Images of a puppy being scolded by his parents. Images of a gray dog barking and breaking things, and being punished. Images of a dog standing still in the corner sadly looking at a white dog and his master eating their meal on a table. Oh, my God! How could I? How could anyone? The man trembled uncontrollably as he wept unashamedly. "God, take me if you will," he sobbed inconsolably, "but first let me make it up to my gray dog."

The man survived his injuries and was let out of the hospital after some days. He took a taxi to his home. As the taxi drove onto his driveway, the dogs heard the noise and ran to the front door. The white dog was ahead of the gray dog as had been their habit for years. The man stepped out of the taxi. The white dog thrashed against the door with full force of his forelegs, in a frenzy of motion. The gray dog peered out from behind the white dog, his whole body heaving with excitement and his tail wagging wildly. The door suddenly gave, spilling the white dog. The dog lunged at his master. The gray dog leaped behind him and then came to an abrupt halt. The man gently pushed the white dog aside, threw his arms wide open, ran toward the gray dog, and hugged him.

The gray dog bit the man.

Why Did the Gray Dog Bite the Man?

There are three possible outcomes of autoregulation. First, there may be the case of an absence of tissue response whereby the individual experiences nothing. Second, the tissues may respond in a positive, comforting way. Third, the tissues may respond in a negative way, the response varying from mild discomfort to severe reactions of intense distress.

Of the three outcomes, the absence of a response is, of course, the easiest to understand. Many people go through life never knowing the energy of life in their tissues. Most of us are not aware of how our tissues can and do respond to us once we have learned how to attend to them. In the prevailing dogma of drug and scalpel medicine, the very concept of tissue response to self-regulatory methods is a taboo subject, fodder for the feeble-minded in medicine. The absence of tissue response supports our notion that only drugs or surgical scalpels are suitable as valid therapies. The possibility of self-regulation for most physicians is a distraction, poorly tolerated because it interferes with our surgical schedules and robs us of the promise of miraculous drug cures.

The second possibility, the tissue energy response, when perceived and experienced by an individual, always brings to him profound insights into the workings of his body organs. The tissues do respond when we learn to attend to them. Of this there can be no doubt. Perceptions of such tissue responses were an integral part of many tribal rituals in earlier times. The ancients understood this phenomenon well. Today, professionals in the biofeedback community accept this as a routine experience for those who practice self-regulation. Every Wednesday in my autoregulation laboratory my patients feel these responses and I demonstrate to them clear electrophysiological changes in the various parts of their bodies that accompany these responses. People describe the positive tissue responses as energy expressed as warmth, flushing, heaviness, magnetic energy, tingling, throbbing or pulsating.

The negative energy responses to self-regulation are just as varied as the positive ones. Many people experience brief episodes of lightheadedness, anxiety, rapid heart rate, discomfort in their eyes with or without watering or searing effects, uneasiness in the chest, mild cramps in the abdomen, spasms in neck muscles and stiffness in low back muscles. In most instances, such responses are of short duration and of no consequence. Almost always, such responses represent a mild expression of symptoms they have suffered in the past. I have observed this phenomenon of pain and suffering arising from simple attempts to still the mind and attend to one's tissues. Why do these tissues do so? Listening to tissues is being kind to them, I reasoned. Why do they protest? Why do they bite back?

The phenomenon of adverse tissue responses ranging from mild discomfort to intense physical suffering has preoccupied me for several years. Why do tissues respond positively sometimes and negatively at others? When tissues do not respond at all, why do they fail to do so? These questions have stayed with me as I have listened to my patients over the years. The stories of the cortical monkey and the limbic dog took shape in my mind as I observed my patients during autoregulation.

THE BITE OF THE NECK MUSCLES

Sheila, a 48-year-old woman, consulted me for sinusitis, chronic headache and fatigue. Following a clinical evaluation and allergy tests, I started some nutritional and allergy therapies. I advised her to get some training in autoregulation methods as I do for all my other patients. She had done some biofeedback previously and was not very eager to consider any other form of self-regulation. Within weeks, her allergy symptoms and headaches improved. After attending my autoregulation workshop, she returned for autoregulation training in our laboratory. I applied the electrodes and other sensors for monitoring her various body functions during autoregulation. After some introductory remarks about what we were going to do, I asked her to sit comfortably on her chair, close her eyes and follow my words.

In autoregulation training, for the first minute or so, I usually observe the subject and his moving graphs on the computer screen and note how cortical or limbic his state of biology is (sharp fluctuations in graph lines with tall peaks and deep valleys indicate cortical turbulence, and smooth and even lines with gentle wave effects reflect a limbic calmness). Sheila visibly stiffened her neck as she closed her eyes, and the computer screen displayed wild fluctuations in her graphs of skin conductance energy, muscle potentials, heart rate and the pulse pressure. This is not unusual for many people and represents apprehension at not knowing what will follow. Generally, such electromagnetic fluctuations subside and I begin to see objective evidence of a transition from a stressful, turbulent cortical state to an even, restorative limbic profile. This was not to be the case with Sheila.

Within several moments, Sheila's neck began to turn and twist. She frowned with closed eyes. Her lips quivered and her jaw muscles tensed up. A few moments later, she broke into clonic, almost convulsive spasms of her twisted neck. To witness sudden, unexpected convulsive activity in a patient who appeared in good health, of course, is not an unusual experience for physicians. I had extensive clinical experience in emergency medicine and surgical trauma cases during my years in surgery and had seen people break out into sudden convulsive activities on many occasions. I am rarely unnerved in clinical settings. This turned out to be an exception. I found Sheila's sudden near-convulsive activity in her twisted neck and her distorted facial features frightening. I suppose because it was the first time I had started out with a patient in a private office setting, very much like someone's living room only to end up abruptly in an emergency. I touched Sheila's hand and asked her to open her eyes. Her clonic neck contractions stopped as suddenly as they had appeared once she'd opened her eyes.

I forced a smile. A faint smile appeared on Sheila's face. We were quiet for a few moments.

"What was that?" I asked, in as natural a tone as I could muster.
"Oh, it's nothing," Sheila replied evenly.

"Nothing?" I asked, surprised at her composure.

"It's nothing. It happens all the time."

"Happens all the time?"

"Yes! I am used to it."

"What is it? How often do you get it? I mean, why didn't you tell me about it?"

"Happens all the time." Sheila forced another smile. "I didn't tell you because I thought there was no point to it."

"No point to it?" I was incredulous.

"No other doctor ever believed me. So I didn't see any point in bothering you with this. I guess the doctors thought it was hysteria or something."

"Maybe it is. Maybe it isn't. Why don't you tell me about it?" I coaxed her.

"Oh! Dr. Ali, there is nothing anyone can do about it. You know it happens every night." Sheila's voice quivered. "Every night, it happens."

I looked at her in silence for a few moments. She looked back at me impassively.

"Tell me more about it." I broke the silence.

"There is nothing more to tell." She shrugged.

"What happens afterward?"

"Every night it happens as I put my head on my pillow and close my eyes. My neck turns and twists and cramps. It hurts me awful." Sheila suddenly broke down and sobbed. I offered her some tissue paper.

"Do you want to stop here?" I said without meaning to say so.

"Not really. When my neck hurts, I open my eyes and the spasms go away. Sometimes I sit up and think. Sometimes I try to read. Then I get exhausted and try again, and again it happens. This goes on all night. Every night."

"When do you sleep?"

"When I am totally exhausted with pain and sleeplessness. Sometimes in the early hours of the morning, maybe four or five, I finally dose off for a few minutes." Sheila sobbed again.

I sat frozen as I listened to her. Tolstoy thought happy people were all alike but each unhappy person was unhappy in his own way. How many Sheilas did he listen to? I wondered. How many Sheilas are there in this world anyway? Living out their lives in silos of sadness.

"Sheila, would you do me a favor?" I asked her, recovering from my personal thoughts. "Would you mind if we did this again?"

"What would that do?" she asked indifferently.

"We might learn something," I encouraged her.

"Learn something?" Sheila smiled again, in earnest, I thought, this time around. "Go ahead, if you think it will help *you*."

I didn't miss her intonation. I hesitated for a minute. Scientific curiosity taking wings at someone else's expense? Now that I write about Sheila I wonder if I knew why I made this request. I knew it was going to distress her again. What did I hope to find? Did I know what might happen? If I did, how did I? It's odd that these questions never arose until now, a few years after that event.

"Yes, Sheila, I think it will help me," I admitted as much.

"Let's do it then," Sheila shrugged her shoulders.

"Can you take the pain if I continue for a few minutes

this time?" I asked.

"Take the pain?" She laughed this time. "What else do I do every night."

"Sheila, this time I am going to close my eyes, too. We will do autoreg together."

We started again. Sheila closed her eyes and the neck contractions returned just as they had the first time. I braced myself, led her into autoregulation again and closed my own eyes. Long hours of autoregulation had given me the ability to turn off my own cortical monkey on rather short notice. I opened my eyes after what seemed to me were five to seven minutes. Sheila's neck still quivered a little, but the intense clonic contractions were gone. Her face appeared calm, her hands resting limp and loose on her thighs. I asked her to open her eyes. We talked for some minutes and then did some more autoregulation. Sheila returned for some more training.

Several months later during a follow-up visit, Sheila told me how her neck problem had mostly cleared except for some nights when she had been extremely stressed after long, demanding hours of work.

Why did Sheila's neck muscles rebel when she closed her eyes? Why did the neck contractions stop when she opened her eyes? And why did the neck muscles finally respond when Sheila and I persisted in listening to them? The purpose of autoregulation, of course, is to comfort the hurt tissues. Why did Sheila's tissues bite back? What possible good, I wondered, did her neck muscles think could come from the games they played? Was it anger turned in as my friends in psychiatry propose? Was it spite? Sheer hostility of the tissues? Did these tissues act so viciously on their own or did they take their cues from somewhere else? Did Sheila's brain send them confusing messages? Was this all mischief perpetrated by the cortical monkey? Or was there a gray dog somewhere? And if there was a gray dog there, why did he bite?

THE BITE OF THE CONFUSED BRAIN CHEMISTRY

Edward ran a profitable engineering company before he was hospitalized for suicidal depression. He suffered from multiple allergies and chemical sensitivities. Prior to and after his hospitalization, Edward consulted a succession of psychiatrists who prescribed almost every single antidepressant described in the Physician Desk Reference. He reacted to all of them except Klonopin, which he took but tolerated poorly. His depression fluctuated widely, and he often became suicidal. His wife, Susan, brought him to me one winter evening. She had learned of my work with nondrug therapies. Susan was hoping, she told me, that diagnosis and management of allergies and chemical sensitivities and nutrient therapies might alleviate some of his depression. All through the first visit, he remained distant and doubtful.

In those early years of my work with environmental medicine and autoregulation, I had the opportunity to care for a large number of patients with allergies and chemical sensitivities who also suffered from depression. Depression in such patients, even when there is a family history of depression, responds well to nondrug management therapies of molecular medicine. None of these patients, however, had been so afflicted with deep, unrelenting depression. I felt inadequate and unsure of my ability to manage such an advanced case. Still, I knew that optimal care of allergies and chemical sensitivities, proper nutritional support and autoregulation could be expected to relieve some of his suffering. My main task, it seemed to me then, was to make sure Edward and his wife understood that. They seemed to understand all this and told me to go ahead. Tentative and uncertain of myself, I proceeded with the examination and micro-elisa allergy tests. In the next visit I reviewed the test results, initiated immunotherapy, prescribed nutrient therapies and gave him training in basic autoregulation. As Susan looked on with evident hope, Edward remained distant and doubtful.

During the next follow-up visit, Edward looked distraught and annoyed. I asked him how he felt.

"You want the truth, Doc?" he asked with unmasked hostility.
"Yes!" I answered.
"I think this whole thing is a hoax," Edward said flatly.
"A hoax?" I was taken aback.
"Yes, a hoax. A hoax to make money," Edward frowned.

Edward's words caught me off guard. This was the first time anyone had accused me in this way. I looked at Susan and fumbled for words. Susan looked embarrassed. I looked out the window for a few brief moments. The sky always has a comforting quality for me.

"Shall we stop here?" I asked Edward as I recovered.
"I don't care. You do what you want to do," he answered

indifferently.

I looked at Susan. She told me they had driven for more than an hour to come to Bloomfield, and asked me if I would continue. Edward simply shrugged his shoulders. Unsure of myself, I proceeded.

A week later, Susan told me Edward was now very intrigued by my basic concept of energy-over-mind — energy of body tissues as the medium of self-regulation. He listened to my tapes, read and re-read *The Cortical Monkey and Healing* and some of my other writings on this subject. His initial doubts appeared to have been replaced with curiosity. He had some problems with alcohol abuse and had attended some meetings of AA and other support groups. He stopped going to those meetings because he had not found them to be very helpful.

The promise of autoregulation, Edward told Susan, was totally different. What appealed to him most was the central idea of autoregulation — of seeking healing with energy, a no-thinking rather than a clever-thinking approach. During one of the early autoregulation training sessions, he had felt pulses in his fingertips and gotten very excited about it, but then it didn't happen again. Still, he persisted with autoregulation.

Days passed and then weeks. Pulses didn't return to his fingertips, nor did any other part of his body respond during autoregulation. Edward read the books again and listened to tapes endlessly. Nothing happened.

The patches of snow on the north side of the woods around our office in Blairstown melted away and bulbs began to sprout. Ground squirrels seemed happy in their spring celebration dance. On many visits, Susan brought along her teenage sons. Strikingly good-looking boys, they made a handsome family, close, loving and full of life — at least that's the way they looked to people who didn't know the deep river of anguish that flowed within them. The boys understood the enormous inner pain of their father and the unending misery of their mom.

Some more weeks passed and Edward continued to suffer, often intensely. He practiced autoregulation regularly, he told me, but there had been no response from any of his tissues. After a few months of persisting, he felt some pulses in his fingertips for a few brief moments in the shower, and then, in his own words, his fingers went dead. I could think of no clear approach. I began to consider the futility of this tack for him. Still, I advised him to persist. His allergy symptoms abated somewhat, but overall there was no appreciable improvement. Hope was fading from Susan's face. Such times are hard on physicians. Would it ever work for Edward? Am I chasing a delusional plausibility? I asked myself.

In late August that year, I conducted a weekend autoregulation workshop for physicians in my office. It seems so improbable now, but I asked Edward if he would attend the workshop. I didn't expect him to understand the highly technical language of my discussion of the energy and molecular basis of the efficacy of autoregulation with my colleagues, but I thought he might have some breakthrough during extended periods of autoregulation practicum during the workshop. Or perhaps, at some deeper, visceral level I was seeking vindication of my therapies that were clearly unproven and could have been easily misconstrued. Edward agreed to come.

Before I began the workshop, I took Edward aside and told him to sit by the back door so he could quietly leave the room if he became uncomfortable at any time during the extended autoregulation exercises. Edward attentively listened to the introductory lectures, though he couldn't hide his frustration at not being able to comprehend the medical jargon. Then we all went into autoregulation and closed our eyes. Within minutes, I sensed some turmoil in the back of the room and opened my eyes to see Edward's back as he hurried out. This is what he told me later when we walked out for lunch:

"Dr. Ali, it was awful! God awful! I closed my eyes and I felt this huge, powerful hand reach down from the darkness above, sharply twist my neck, and try to yank my head through the ceiling. I just had to get out. I'm sorry, Dr. Ali. I am very sorry. I know what you are trying to do. But it's no use."

FIELDS OF CANDLES

Depression is a problem of confused brain chemistry, I tried to explain to Edward when I saw him after the fiasco at the physician meeting. I told him to imagine that there was a field of candles. Below the surface all of the candles were wired. When the winds blew, many of those candles were put out. The circuitry connecting the candles beneath the surface came to life and lit the extinguished candles. It all happened in moments. No one realized that one candle had gone out. No one, of course, who had intact circuitry.

When cells are hit hard by injurious elements, be they chemical injuries to nerve cells or sad thoughts that deplete the energy neurotransmitters at the cell membranes, the cells recover, largely because they *network*. Cells knew about networking long before the yuppie generation did when it got laid off after the stock market crash. The candles in the cells are lit up by electromagnetic matchsticks sent to them by their friendly neighbor cells.

It is different with people who suffer from depression. Their cells crave for the day (adrenergic) and night (serotinergic) neurotransmitters, but the neurotransmitters are nowhere to be found. Their network connections are weak, sometimes moribund, near death. When the winds blow, they put out the candles. The cells in the neighborhood watch helplessly. Then there are yet more winds and yet more candles go out. And it goes on and on till, as one patient who suffers from depression and who listened to me talk about the fields of candles put it, there are no more lit candles. There is darkness of deep depression. Deep holes that sink deeper and deeper. And then there are no walls around the holes. Only a free fall into abysmal darkness.

I told Edward I had seen people learn how to banish those winds of the thinking mind when they first feel them rising. I had seen what the limbic tissue energy can do. I had seen all that through the eyes of my patients who had been there. There, deep in those dark recesses. I also wondered where the true hope ended and deception began. I wondered if the experience of these other people had any relevance to Edward.

I don't know why and how Edward persisted with

autoregulation. Some months later, disillusioned with the results, I suggested to Edward and Susan that they consult some other physicians who might have better luck than I did. "Doc, you want to throw me out, do it. I am not going to see any more doctors. I have seen enough for one lifetime," Edward answered emphatically.

It took Edward several months before he began to sense the response from his tissues with autoregulation. He told me he was able to do things at home and sometimes at work, and didn't much think about the relief that death might bring anymore. My notes written on Edward's chart next summer include the following quotation from Susan, "After nineteen years, Edwards has lived this summer." I was deeply moved by her words. Edward followed it by telling me how successfully he was coping with heavy, ongoing losses at his business and how he was dealing with the possibility of declaring bankruptcy.

"Doc, it is hard to believe I am doing all this and still continue to think of the future of my family," he told me one day.

How much can a person take? No one knows enough to be a pessimist, Cousins' words came to me. There is a limit, an absolute limit to how much anyone can suffer, came the response from within me. What can he do to absorb these new shocks? I wondered. I advised Edward to consider joining the local Recovery chapter in his area and attend their group meetings. Now that his body was beginning to respond, I told Edward, it might be of great value for him to attend Recovery meetings. Edward and Susan listened to me intently.

"Doc, you are a very funny man," Edward's face broke

into a broad grin.

"What did I say that's so funny?" I asked, somewhat overwhelmed by his sudden outburst of energy.

"You are funny! Doc, very funny," he went on as his wife looked at him with obvious confusion.

"Yes! I am funny, Edward. But I still do not know what you found so funny?" I spoke plaintively.

"Doc! How could you tell me to go to Recovery group meetings?"

"Because I think folks at Recovery are very good at what they do," I answered matter-of-factly.

"Doc, you forget what I told you when I first saw you. Remember I told you I had been to AA and several church groups. I told you the talking therapies had not worked for me. You are the one who first told me to try the tissue energy approach. You are the one who first talked to me about listening to tissues. Perceiving their energy as you call it. Enhancing it. And when the tissues wouldn't talk back to me, you told me to hang on. So I hung on. Boy, did I hang on! I bought all that. And now that things are beginning to shape up, you tell me to return to those group meetings. You are funny! Doc, you are a very funny man." Edward stopped talking and looked at me as if he had just swallowed a canary.

****

Why did Edward's abnormal brain chemistry bite him so hard as he closed his eyes? The cortical monkey again? Or was there something more to that? Was it an ugly prank of the monkey, or a painful bite of the dog?

Why did the gray dog bite his master anyway? Was he angry? Vengeful? What did he want? Revenge for all the years of neglect, of hurt, of absence of love? How could he have known what had passed before his master's eyes in the hospital intensive care unit? How could he have known what his master felt that day? How could he have known he was going to be hugged that day? Had he been scheming silently for years for that day to arrive? So he could bite him and get even for years of suffering? How could he have figured all that in that one brief moment when the man brushed aside his beloved white dog and ran to him? Or was the gray dog simply confused? Did the man's hug stun the limbic dog in him? Did the limbic dog suddenly get disoriented by an unexpected burst of love? Love coming from someone he thought incapable of loving him? Why then? Why not on some earlier day?

Why did the limbic dog bite?

DO MOLECULES, CELLS AND TISSUES HAVE CONSCIOUSNESS?

Do tissues have consciousness? I am told what separates man from the beast is consciousness. Man, such reasoning goes, is capable of rational thought; hence, he is rational. Where do human tissues fit in? With man, the rational being, or with the beast, the living thing without any consciousness? Are human tissues mere globs of protoplasm? Without consciousness? Ugly clumps of cells, blood and tissue fluid? Heaps of shining insignificance? So what are human tissues? Confused dogs, ready to bite? They cannot be trusted anytime, anywhere without the constant censor of the thinking head. The cortical monkeys look away for a passing moment and the limbic dogs bite!

I do not know much about the consciousness that the enthusiasts of artificial intelligence talk about. Those who profess to understand consciousness and seek to relate it to the artificial intelligence of computers, it seems to me, are simply putting on airs. Nor do I understand the basis of the recent claim of Crick and Koch that the "problem of consciousness" is on the verge of solution (*Scientific American* September 1992). But I do know this: The injured tissues do not lie. The only part of the human condition that lies to us is the thinking brain. The heart, the lungs, the kidneys, muscles, tendons and the skin never learned to lie. When we do choose to listen to the injured tissues, they do speak the truth. This is the truth about the language of injured tissues. This is the truth about the bite of the limbic dog. How do I know? Because I know the limbic dog is not into biting. The limbic dog is a loving dog. Sheila found out. So did Edward. I know of hundreds of Sheilas and Edwards who found this out.

If bad thoughts can cause cancer, I heard an expert pronounce on the radio some time ago, why can't good thoughts make it go away? The expert then went on to congratulate himself for the clarity of his thoughts. I wondered if this expert had ever really cared for anyone with cancer. He is right about the first part of his discovery. Indeed, unrelenting bad thoughts can create relentless stress that can break our molecular and energy defenses, and so lead to production of tumors. How does this expert know that the tumor cells — or for that matter healthy cells — care about our infatuation with our thoughts, and the notions that our thoughts metamorphose into the physical reality of our choosing. My patients have taught me that *tissues respond only when we attend to them in a no-thinking mode.* Tissues do not seem to care much about our great intellectual prowess. They have little respect for our clever intellectual schemes.

I see many patients who tell me they can control their migraine headaches and asthma attacks with mind control. Someone once told me he even "killed" his cancer by turning off its blood supply. This always fascinates me. I do not for a single moment doubt that they are telling me the truth as *they* see it. So I ask them to explain how they use their minds to control their headaches or asthma attacks. This is how the conversations have gone many times.

"Tell me, how do you control your asthma attack?" I ask.

"By mind control," the patient replies.

"Good! Now, tell me how do you do mind control?" I ask again.

"By mind-over-body," the patient repeats.

"That's good. How do you do your mind-over-body thing?" I repeat myself.

"You know how! By mind-over-body."

"That's really wonderful. Now tell me how do you do it?"

"By ... By mind over ..."

"Yes, I know it is by mind-over-body. But tell me how you do it," I persist. "I write about this stuff. I can't write mind-over-body over and over again, can I?"

There is usually a long pause. Then comes a hesitant answer:

"I guess I really don't know. But honest, Doc, it has happened many times," he speaks defensively.

"Of course, it has happened many times," I reassure him.

I believe him. I have no valid reason to call his assertion a lie or consider it a delusional plausibility. I do, however, have a strong sense that the asthma attack subsides not because he has figured out a clever way to send some clever electromagnetic impulses from his thinking cortical brain to the tightened muscles in his bronchial tubes. Rather, by some great intuitive insight he has learned to keep his cortical monkey out of the way of his bronchial tubes. Delivered from the ceaseless chatter of the mind, the limbic muscles in the bronchi tube open up. They do so because that's what they were designed to do. The bronchial muscles do not know how to write computer software. Neither do they know how to read poetry. They open up because that's the only thing they know how to do. The thinking mind can shut them off, but it doesn't know how to open them up. That they must do by themselves, by some limbic quality, without any help from the cortical monkey.

THE BITE OF THE PSYCHONEUROIMMUNE DOG

Tammy, a woman in her late forties, consulted me for multiple sclerosis. She had experienced abnormal sensations in her limbs with "pins and needles" and weakness of muscles for a few months. She became very frightened when she started losing her balance and had difficulty walking. MRI scans ordered by one neurologist showed demyelinating lesions in her brain and spinal cord. A second MRI scan ordered by a second neurologist confirmed the diagnosis of multiple sclerosis.

"I know it's not that," Tammy spoke after I finished reading her file and looked up.

"It's not what?" I asked, without really needing any clarification of her words.

"It's not multiple sclerosis," she said firmly.

"How do you know?"

"I just know."

"How?" I persisted.

"Because that's what happened the last time," she replied emphatically.

"What happened last time?"

"They said it was lupus and they gave me cortisone. I threw the cortisone out after a few weeks."

"Then what?"

"Then I took a lot of vitamins and my lupus went away."

"How was lupus diagnosed," I asked, feigning surprise.

"They did all the tests. ANA, LE prep and a test for proteins in the urine. You know, everything the rheumatologists do."

I had gotten used to such stories by then. The first few times had been different. It had been hard to believe patients who told me such stories. It literally meant throwing out all my medical texts. Patients with serious autoimmune disorders such as lupus and multiple sclerosis are not supposed to get better by simply taking vitamin pills, at least not according to our medical texts. The hard-nosed pathologist in me had great difficulty in believing what medical texts said couldn't be believed. Then things changed for me. My patients forced me to think differently. With the passing years, I saw too many patients who'd positive lupus and rheumatoid factor tests go on to recover and lived healthy lives for years. I realized the tests simply indicate signals of stresses on our immune defenses. Nothing more. How many times does one have to be hit on his head?

"Tell me something about the stress in your life." I returned from my own thoughts.

"You know how it is. Everyone suffers stress in life," she replied.

"That's true. Still, tell me. Is he very supportive?" I asked her, gesturing to her husband who had sat silently listening to us.

"Yeah, he is supportive," she replied after a slight initial hesitation.

We physicians do learn with time. Minor delays in answers often tell us more than many carefully crafted answers from our patients. I smiled at her husband and returned to my questions.

"What was the year they told you had lupus?" I asked.

"1984." Tammy leaned back in the chair.

"What happened in '84?"

"Nothing!"

"What happened in '83?"

"Nothing!"

"Nothing in '84 and nothing in '83?" I looked into her eyes, persisting in my inquiry.

"What happened in 83?" Tammy sat up.

"Yes, what happened in 83?"

"My mother died." Tammy's neck stiffened.

"Were you close?"
"Very."
"Very close?"
"She was my best friend."
"What happened early this year?"
"What do you mean?"
"What happened in the months before you developed pins and needles in legs and arms?"

A hurt expression crossed Tammy's face and she sat up. I looked at her in silence. She seemed to read my mind and quickly recovered her composure. Then she turned her face to her husband who glanced at me uncomfortably. I looked back at Tammy.

"We had family troubles."
"Would you rather not talk about them?" I asked.
"No! There is nothing to hide. We separated for some months."
"And then?"
"Then we got together to see if we could make it."
"And then?"
"And then we realized it had to end. There had to be a divorce."

Tammy broke down. I didn't have to look at her husband to learn anything more. Was there a chance for some wound healing there? I wondered. Serious illnesses sometimes break good marriages. Sometimes they also mend broken ones. If the latter was going to prevail, it would not be the first time I had seen a major disease lead to healing of deep wounds of lost love. Those things just seem to happen.

"Tell me, how do you react to perfumes and formaldehyde and tobacco smoke?" I changed the subject. Tammy slumped back into the chair.

Psychoneuroimmunology, my friends who thrive on the matters of mind and body tell me, is the branch of medicine that deals with interrelationships between the psyche, nervous system and the immune system. It is a jaw breaker of a word. Whenever anyone throws this term at me, my thoughts go to Socrates and his oft-quoted words:

The great error of our day is this: Our physicians separate mind from body.

It fascinates me. It took us about two centuries of medical research to separate the mind from the body. It took us a near century to define the immune system as a system of antibodies and antigens, quite discrete from the brain and our psyche. And now we are devoting hundreds of thousands of hours in research and spending millions of dollars to prove that these indeed are interrelated. We physicians excel in reinventing the wheel. Old Socrates, he had the last laugh.

How did Tammy's immune system turn against her? How did the loss of her mother lead to the formation of antibodies against the nuclei of her own cells — that is what ANA (anti-nuclear antibodies) are. Eight years later, how did the threatened loss of her husband turn her immune system against her own myelin sheaths? Myelin sheaths are the insulation cover of nerves that normally prevent short-circuiting of electromagnetic impulses passing through the nerves. That is the essence of multiple sclerosis. What did the death of Tammy's mother have to do with her developing lupus? What did her impending divorce have to do with her myelin sheaths? Why did the psychoneuroimmune animal in Tammy bite her?

Perhaps some day we will have a better understanding of the healing energy of God. Then we will be able to answer the obvious questions with the objectivity demanded by science. For now, I am convinced tissues, cells, molecules and electrons have their own intelligence, their own consciousness. They *feel and respond.* As for the purist in science who feels a surging desire to ridicule me, I ask only that he observe individual cells shaved from living tissues and kept in tissue culture petri dishes. Observe and reflect upon the greater glory of the intelligence and consciousness of these cells. Reflect on how they adapt to their new life in the petri dish. See with awe the sheer energy of life.

I ask the skeptic in medicine to consider nitric oxide. It is a simple gas made up of an atom of nitrogen and oxygen each. It is a triumph of nature in molecular design, a marvel of biology. One of the simplest compounds known to us, nitric oxide is elegance in simplicity. It opens up the arteries thrown into spasms by adrenaline and its companions in cortical conspiracies. Tight arteries are tired arteries. They scream for help. An enzyme, nitric oxide synthase, acts upon amino acid arginine and splits a molecule of nitric oxide, leaving behind molecules of another amino acid, citrulline. It is this simple molecule of nitric oxide that also serves as a messenger, whereby immune cells called phagocytes recognize and destroy foreign invaders like disease-causing bacteria and errant cells that cause cancer.

The nitric acid molecule fascinates me because it makes sense where nothing else does. It is produced by individual cells in times of their need — without any commands from the thinking mind. Nitric acid production is a local energy event. Each nitric acid molecules produced locally in response to a *local* need puts to a lie the common belief that clever thinking — mind-over-body approach — heals. This simple molecule gives me a rational, scientifically sound and believable chemical and energy mechanism to help me comprehend — partially at best — how autoregulation works in real life. It helps explain why autoregulation does not work for some people for long months, and how it does work when finally it does. This molecule is one of those that hold the key to understanding how exhausted tissues may — and do — finally escape the cortical tunnels and walk onto limbic openness. And, yes, it does open some windows to Sheila's suffering. And the suffering of Edward and Tammy. And of the suffering of all the other Sheilas and Edwards and Tammys. Nitric oxide, of course, is not a lone warrior rising against adrenergic tyranny. There are others. Some of them we know. Some others, I am sure, will be recognized at some future time.

THE BITE OF ADRENERGIC HYPERVIGILENCE

A man gambles and his wife suffers from diarrhea. A man fears he will lose his job after 25 years of work with his company. A woman cares for her mother dying of cancer and suffering from unremitting pain. A salesman returns home without a sale and weary with fatigue. We say they live in stress.

A young man suffers a sudden panic attack. He cannot breathe, has heart palpitations and thinks he is dying of a heart attack. A woman dashes into the street to yank away her toddler who is walking toward a speeding car. A leopard chases a deer and the deer sprints to dodge the attacker. What are the molecular dynamics of these events? Chemistry of the stress reaction, the so-called fight or flight response. The role of adrenaline and its cousin molecules, catecholamines, in the cause of stress is well-known. In the stress reaction, arteries in limbs and abdominal organs tighten, muscles in the body tense up, pupils dilate, heart rate quickens, skin rises in goose pimples, and the cortical brain shifts to a higher gear. Nature gave us this reaction for a survival advantage, so we can escape faster to safety or dig our heels to fight out the aggressor for life. The problem is these cortical molecular devices do not know their limits. Once triggered, they initiate cascade events, forever feeding upon themselves.

The so-called chronic stress syndrome, of course, is nothing but adrenergic molecular hypervigilence. In this syndrome, the body organs are hit hard with a new stressor before they have a chance to recover from the previous insult. Relentless stress causes unrelenting demands on body organs; the tissues scramble, suffer and finally suffocate. The role of many other neurotransmitters in the cause of other chronic disorders has been expounded in recent studies. The common thread in the energy dynamics in all these states is *cortical overdrive*. The question that has preoccupied me for some years is this: How do tissues counter cortical molecular hypervigilence? How do they escape from cortical torrents? How do they return to a limbic state? Do they do so because the cortical brain sends electromagnetic messages to them to ease up? Or does it send some neurotransmitters to cancel out the effects of adrenaline and its companion molecules in cortical conspiracies? Or do individual cells in tightened arteries and spastic muscles have their own molecular devices to escape the tyranny of cortical tyrants?

How do adrenergic dogs bite? In the same way a teenager jolts his car on his first driving lesson. Letting go in comfort and peace does not come the way a meal comes at a fast food outlet. Molecules have their own rhythms, their own timing, their own sense of space.

Every Wednesday I give autoregulation training to a group of four or five new patients. I hear the moans of a limbic dog in one or two patients in almost each group. Fortunately, the bite of the limbic dog is not as bad for most people as it was for Sheila and Edward and Tammy. Most people experience spasms in their neck muscles, low back stiffness, mild chest discomfort, anxiety, rapid heart rate, lightheadedness, and occasional episodes of watering or searing eyes. Such limbic bites are brief and of no consequnece. All a person has to do to overcome them is to persist in autoregulation.

There is a cortical monkey in each one of us. Most of us see him clearly. There is a limbic dog in each one of us. Many of us are totally oblivious of his existence.

I end this chapter with a few sentences with which I ended *The Cortical Monkey and Healing*:

"It seems improbable that man will ever fully understand the healing energy of love, or to be more precise, the healing energy of God. Medical technology, itself an expression of God's energy, is beginning to allow us to measure some things about love, and then reproduce them. Measurements and reproducibility make up the language of science. One day, it seems to me, the men of medicine and men of spirits will meet at some summit of union. The energy of love will have brought them together."

" ... often we look so long at the closed door that we do not see the one that has been opened before us."

Helen Keller

Chapter 2

The Ghoraa and Limbic Running

The Limbic Principle of Exercise

The limbic principle of exercise combines exercise with a deeply personal, treasured time of meditation and silence. Several observations, some personal, many related to me by others, led to the shaping of this principle in my mind over many years.

One of my early memories relates to a trip that I took with my father and brothers when I was eight or nine. We left Dera Ghazi Khan, a town in western Pakistan, to visit a village in the country, a 60-mile long trip. We were traveling along a dirt road over dry, hilly, wilderness terrain, which at times turned into a desert. It was a hot summer day. The wind blew as if it came out of a furnace. Every now and then we saw a camel cart along the way and some goats and sheep in the distance. That was about it. For miles we didn't see any villages or people.

Sometime during the afternoon, our car broke down. The road was deserted. The afternoon breeze began to cool us down. In the afternoon, the desert wilderness loses its harshness and becomes kind and hospitable. Living things in the desert, paralyzed by the blistering heat of the noontime sun, come back to life with the cool evening breeze. We waited for an hour or so for some bus, truck or car to come along so we could hitch a ride. No luck. My brothers and I didn't mind it very much. It was not an unpleasant break for us. We walked around, picked up stones and threw them aimlessly. Soon the sun went down.

My father was a session judge who spent most of his time trying murder cases. He worked hard at dispensing British colonial justice to the tribal Baluchi people. The Baluchi didn't care much for the British justice code. They followed their own Jurga system of justice: They simply killed off whoever didn't subscribe to their point of view about tribal justice. They remembered some things well but had a very poor memory for others. That meant my father had to frequently play sleuth. He often traveled to distant villages to study the murder sites and to talk to people who didn't recall certain things well. He figured he had a better chance to learn the facts while sitting in their mud houses, the facts they surely wouldn't remember in his court. While walking those long distances, he would often recite Quranic (from the Koran) verses.

My father decided we would continue walking to the village and keep hoping for some ride to come along. I asked my father how long the walk was going to be. He answered 11 or 12 miles. I asked him how much that was. One fourth of the way, he answered. That hit me like a rock. We had traveled all day long, it seemed to me. If that was three fourths of the way, then the next one fourth was going to be a long walk, a very long walk. I was hungry by now. We had no food with us. That meant it was going to be a long, hungry walk. There was nothing to be seen on the way. It would soon be very dark and desolate.

My father began to recite verses from the Quran. We started the walk. I kept looking back, hoping to see a car or a truck. There was nothing to be seen. Not even some goats or sheep. Only a thin line of a road disappearing into the distance. Nevertheless, my father's face was peaceful. There was not a trace of strain on it. He obviously enjoyed his recital of Quranic

---

verses. (He was limbic, though I didn't fully understand this in those early days.) My father knew in those days that nobody traveled at night on dirt roads in the wilderness. I was not told that until the next morning.

After walking a few hundred yards, my brothers and I became tired. Every few minutes one of us asked my father how much distance we had covered and how much of it was left behind. My father replied with a smile sometimes, but stayed absorbed in his verses at other times. When he didn't answer, we didn't get angry because he was not one of those individuals people got angry with often. At least I don't remember ever getting angry at my father. (Years later I would realize what it means for someone never to be angry at his father.)

Sometime during that walk (after an interminable count of hills and valleys in the road, it seemed to me) I stopped and firmly demanded that my father tell me exactly how long it was going to be and why he could not arrange things better. He stopped his recital and looked at me tenderly. "We are all going to recite from the Quran now. We will all take turns reciting and we will recite until we reach the village. Then, when we get there, we will eat our meals and go to sleep," he said in an even, soft tone. He asked my eldest brother to start the recitation.

I don't remember much of what transpired after that. I *do* remember that I recited many Quranic verses during those hours. I have a clear memory of reaching the village and sleeping on a bed with lily-white bed sheets. No, I do not remember if I was very hungry then. Nor do I remember if my legs ached from walking long miles. Nor if my feet hurt with blisters. Nor if I had asked my father many questions about the distance after we had started the verses.

This trip often comes back to me when I write or talk about going limbic. Going limbic! I wonder how much this early memory of a trip with my father has to do with my concepts and practice of limbic methods that evolved many years later.

THE GHORAA RUN

As far as I know, ghoraas pulling tongas over long distances run limbically.

Kirto is my ancestral village in Pakistan. During my childhood, the only way to reach Kirto was by a tonga [a poor man's buggy pulled by a ghoraa (horse)]. Kirto is located about three miles from Narang, a small town on the railroad track which links the city of Lahore, where I went to medical school, to the town of Sialkot, where Talat (my beautiful wife) went to school. During my childhood, we often took the slow passenger train from Lahore to Narang, and then took a tonga trip to Kirto. The tonga traveled along a bumpy dirt road with wide, open rice paddies on both sides of the road. It often passed through mud ditches. Often the passengers were asked to get out and walk across the ditch. Sometimes the mud was too thick for the ghoraa pulling the tonga, and the passengers were required to push the tonga. The ride often took us an hour and a half for the three-mile distance.

The tonga wallas (drivers) made a meager living. They often severely overloaded their tongas to increase their profits. While the tongas were designed for four adults, they often loaded 10 or 12 children and adults. We children were asked to sit, stand or simply hang on to one or another part of the tonga. I have many vivid memories of some of those tonga trips. Squeezed hard among other passengers, sometimes my view was restricted to just one part of the ghoraa. There were days when I didn't much care to look at the only part of the ghoraa's anatomy which was available for my viewing. Sometimes I got to watch the ghoraa's head, which was a treat.

Ghoraas harnessed in tongas have *khoppas* (large, ugly, curved pieces of dried, shriveled leather) tied over their eyes. There is an awful lot a young boy, packed tight on a tonga within a heap of passengers, can wonder about if all he can see on a long tonga trip is the head of a blindfolded ghoraa. How does a blindfolded ghoraa run for long periods of time? What does he think about? How does he know the distance he has to go? How does he know how far he has come? How does he know how much farther he has to go? What part of his body gets tired first? How does he rest that part? Or does he? The ghoraa must want to rid himself of the harness. How often does he do that? But he does not succeed. How does he put up with that? Why doesn't he get angry? And if he does, why doesn't he show it? Does he ever become sad? How sad does he become? And when he is sad, who does he talk to about his sadness?

I observed those ghoraas for hours. There were endless questions. I would think of the answers. Then I would reject my first answers and start thinking of new ones. Sometimes I thought the ghoraa knew what I was thinking about and wanted to give me the real answers. But then there would be the loud curse of the tonga walla and the jolting sound of the whip and the ghoraa would move his legs faster. That would usually do it. For some time I would lose my interest and my mind would wander.

Don't the khoppas bother the ghoraa? I mean, it must be very annoying for the ghoraa not to be able to see. See where he is going and who is coming from where he is going? What is it that khoppas do anyway, blind the ghoraa? Obviously that does happen. But is that all? So why do ghoraas tolerate khoppas? Why don't they rip them apart? Ghoraa don't have hands, but I see them do all kinds of funny things with their teeth. Certainly they could help each other in this.

At times I was convinced the ghoraa pulling the tonga wasn't there. Oh, he was there physically, but *he was not there.* The tonga walla talked incessantly to the passengers. The ghoraa simply ran. He did not look ahead or around. He was oblivious to the world around him or the tonga behind him. His legs moved with a rhythm of their own. His head bobbed up and down. His neck swung with gentle to and fro motions. His shoulder muscles dropped a little rhythmically with each step. His torso seemed to float along. The hoofs hit the soft ground and raised little billows of dirt. The ghoraa simply ran. There was no judgment. There was no anger. There was no sense of captivity. There was no resentment. There was no right way of running and no wrong way of running. Only running. The ghoraa simply ran.

Rug Running

I spend the bulk of my daily morning exercise time on a custom-made "treadmill." This treadmill is actually a piece of rug, three feet by three feet, and my treadmill running is what I call rug-running (running in place on a rug). After many experiments with running on the track, beach and other locations, I find my rug-running most conducive to limbic running. The small rug serves as an anchor for me.

When I first started limbic running, it was not unusual for me to feel some heaviness or resistance in my legs. Muscle stretching relieved this to a large degree, but it still persisted. Within minutes, the muscles would loosen up, breathing would slow down, hands would begin to throb and pulsate, and I would be well on my way. Minutes flew by. I moved to my jump rope routine and some more stretches. Then I came to my rug-running.

My pattern of limbic exercise has not changed since my early days of research with limbic breathing and limbic exercise. The difference is that now there is no initial resistance from my leg muscles. Just minutes after beginning, my breathing slows even further. My eyelids begin to droop, and often my eyes close spontaneously. I sometimes open my eyes, but the eyes close again. There is gray openness all around me. Some more time passes by. Then there is light all around me. I escape into this light of limbic openness. I lose sense of time. Such limbic rug-running continues until I pull myself out.

Now I look forward to this deeply personal time each morning. A time without cortical clutter, without cortical greed, without cortical scheming and without my cortical monkey on my back. Only limbic gratitude and limbic openness exist.

Coming out of a limbic exercise (I call it "limbic break"), I often see things in new ways. It was in such moments that I saw a ghoraa running. He was simply running — running the way I used to see them in my childhood. There were khoppas on his eyes. The ghoraa made no effort. He simply ran. His legs moved with their own rhythm. His loin muscles quivered with low, rhythmic motions. His head bobbed up and down. His neck moved gently to and fro. His shoulders dropped a little with each step. His torso floated along. He didn't seem to care where he was coming from, nor where he might be going. There was no concern about the length of the run. No eagerness to reach the end of the run. No anger. No sadness. Simple running. *Is this limbic running?* I wondered. Is that how the ghoraas run when they are harnessed in tongas? Limbically? Is that why they do not look angry, hostile or sad?

THE KHOPPA EFFECT

What do khoppas have to do with this? As a child I had wondered why the ghoraas didn't violently protest khoppas and why the tonga wallas used them in the first place. Now after my own run with closed eyes, I wondered about the khoppa effect in a different light. Do khoppas help the ghoraas keep their cortical monkeys away? Do the ghoraas go limbic? Do khoppas help the ghoraas escape into their limbic openness? Is it the same thing as closing my eyes to escape into my limbic openness?

Why do we close our eyes during prayers, or during meditation, or during periods of sudden joy and intense pain? Why does a Japanese close his eyes in a crowded Tokyo subway car? How did the primitive man learn the value of closing his eyes? Is it just to cancel out the visual perceptions, as we are told, or is there a deeper, more spiritual purpose behind this? In all cultures, in all societies and in all regions of the world, people close their eyes on many occasions and for many ceremonies. If asked why, they are likely to shrug their shoulders. But they *know* the answer at some deeper inner level.

The act of closing the eyes, it seems to me, has a lot to do with inner calm, a visceral stillness that I call the Khoppa Effect. It is through this Khoppa Effect that we come to be conscious of the larger *presence* to which I alluded in my description of limbic openness earlier in this chapter. It is the Khoppa Effect that liberates us from our compulsion to measure, analyze and define the universe around us in *our* terms. The Khoppa Effect brings us the gift of limbic gratitude and frees us from the cortical greed. We then accept the link between us and the larger *presence* around us. The awareness and the consciousness of this link may be all that we can ever achieve.

Two simple observations may be cited here. The first concerns the stressors acting on the mind. Eyes receive more noxious information than any other body organ. We see stressors much more than we hear them, taste them or feel them. The second has to do with the stressors on our biologic responses. Referred pain comes to the eyes from more muscles than any other body organ (orbicularis and other periorbital muscles, masseter and other facial muscles, frontalis and other forehead muscles, sternomastoid and other neck muscles, trapezius and other back muscles, and temporalis and other scalp muscles). These two observations explain why many patients with depression, anxiety and related disorders often find their suffering most intensely expressed in their eyes.

Man has known and used the Khoppa Effect for eons, in different ways, for different reasons, and with different results. The enormous benefits of closing one's eyes, partly or completely, during a limbic exercise is but one small expression of the Khoppa Effect.

THE AFRICAN TRIBAL MESSAGE CARRIER

The accounts of African tribal message carriers fascinate me. These men run barefoot on hot sand under a blazing sun for as many as fifty miles. When they reach their destination and deliver their messages, they don't pant for breath. They do not hyperventilate. They do not perspire. They do not suffer from any heart palpitations. They are not dehydrated. They run in the wilderness and the wilderness is their companion. The dirt under their feet, the bush around their path, the open sky above them. And yes, the openness all around them. The

African message runners run limbically. In what sort of physiologic state are they? Are they in the same state in which our mice or medical students are when they are put on treadmills? Certain levels of performance are demanded of our mice and medical students by those who conduct such experiments with them. Who demands what of the tribal message runners?

Our laboratory mice and medical students run to the ugly humming of our treadmills as they eye the syringes that our researchers hold ready to plunge into their flesh to retrieve their blood samples. Blood darkened by the strain of machines that jolt them with their noises, computers that flash at them their ominous signals, and the professionals who unnerve them with their sharp, doubting eyes.

What do these mice and medical students have in common with the African tribal message carriers? The tribal man runs to the calling of some distant drummers, in harmony with the nourishing Mother Earth and the open, loving sky. To whose tune do the poor mice and medical students march? These are the "research" studies by which we are asked to live our lives.

PEOPLE WITH A LIGHT FOOT

Tarahumaras, the Indians living in the Chihuahua mountains of northern Mexico, call themselves the "Rar'amuri," meaning The People with a Light Foot. Their favorite sport is long-distance running, 100 or more miles at a time. Carl Lumholtz, the Norwegian explorer, wrote about a Tarahumara Indian who ran over 600 miles in five days in desert country (without Pegasus running shoes). How did the Tarahumaras run? By reaching the 70th percentile of their maximum heart rate? By counting their breathing rate? By thinking about how they were lowering their LDL cholesterol? Or raising their HDL cholesterol? Were they looking for endorphin "highs"?

Limbic running is running with light feet. Tarahumaras were not into running. They were into the joys of life that came to them through their light feet. Tarahumaras were into limbic running. They must have known something about limbic openness, for limbic openness is a universal human experience, except for those totally consumed by their cortical impulses.

THE GAS STATION THAT WASN'T THERE

Akbar Naeem, M.D., my roommate in medical school, visited me recently. He used to run for fitness, now he does NordicTrack at home. We talked about the physiology of running. He related the following experience:

"I was running late one evening, when I saw a gas station. This was my usual route, and I knew this gas station did not exist. So where did it come from? I became puzzled. Did I lose my way? Am I confused? I looked around. The street was my street. What is this, a syncope attack? For one brief moment, I was frightened. I looked around one more time. It was the right street. How did the gas station materialize there? Then I realized what had happened. I thought I had just begun my run, when in reality I was close to the finish. I was used to seeing the gas station at the end of the run and not at the beginning. It seems I had completed my three mile run without knowing that I had done so."

The preceding is a perfect illustration of what limbic running is all about. Dr. Naeem ran limbically, though the word limbic would have meant nothing to him at that time.

Limbic running is not about marking time. It is not about measuring distance. It is not about planning for the day. It is not about "going over yesterday's activity." It is not about "working out our problems."

Limbic running is about listening to our tissues. It is about perceiving the energy in them. It is about being kind to ourselves. It is about escaping into limbic stillness. It is about limbic openness. And, yes, it is about a link with *that* larger presence which is always with us.

FIFTEEN LIMBIC MINUTES

To Dr. Naeem's story, I add one of my own. One morning I woke up to the realization that my associate pathologist, Evalynne Braun, M.D., might not be able to come to the hospital early enough to cover our frozen-section service for patients requiring biopsy diagnosis during their operations. She had suffered from one of her migraine attacks the day before and that usually leaves her exhausted. My other associate pathologist, Verna Atkins, M.D., was away on vacation. I looked at my watch and realized that I might not be able to do my usual half hour of limbic running.

I rose from my bed, did my stretching exercises, took my nutrient supplements with water, pulled my watch out and walked out to the patio for my usual rug-running. There I looked at my watch, decided to run for 15 minutes, put my watch on the floor and started my run. When it occurred to me that it might be 15 minutes since I started running, I looked at my watch. My watch told me a different story. I had been running for 32 minutes.

There are two principal reasons people do not exercise: inertia and boredom. There is only one solution: Make exercise time a deeply personal time for inner visceral stillness. This was the insight that the 15 limbic minutes brought me.

LEGS HURT WITH STRAIGHT TOES

One of my physician colleagues related to me the following story. He took up jogging. Within a few weeks, the initial muscle aches subsided and he became comfortable at it. One day he thought of consulting a coach to improve his running technique. The coach conducted what he called computerized stride analysis with video equipment and concluded that my friend did not run with straight toes. The coach explained how even one inch off from the straight line means loss of distance covered, that each inch of distance lost with each step matters, and that it all adds up. The coach then proceeded to instruct my friend in the proper technique of running with straight toes. My friend was excited by this insight. He pursued the *correct* method of running with straight toes. Within a few days his legs started to hurt during his runs. This problem persisted until my friend decided to quit jogging altogether. He wondered about what might have caused the pain in his legs. Weeks later it occurred to him that the leg pain may indeed have something to do with his straight toe running. He resumed his natural way of jogging. The pain didn't return.

Again, to this I add one of my own experiences. During

my research for writing this book I experimented with many different ways of exercise. I ran in the park and on the street, on the track and on the beach. I experimented with the 70th percentile and the 85th percentile (that is how I know how irrelevant and meaningless such "science" of exercise is to our well-being and health). All during this rather prolonged period of experimentation I was extremely careful not to put undue stress on my ligaments, tendons and muscles. I diligently avoided missteps and sprained joints. Still, I developed aches and pains in different parts of my body at different times, never really knowing how and when I injured my tissues. This never happens to me when I do limbic running.

How often have I seen my colleagues spiritedly talk about their running programs at lunchtime? How often do I see them limp around the hospital wards after some weeks or months? How often does exercise become a regular part of their day? How often does it become a period of personal time, not for computing their lowered LDL cholesterol values, their raised HDL cholesterol values and their reduced lipid coronary risk ratios? With some exceptions, sore backs and sprained ankles announce the demise of their great initiatives, casualties of the cortical monkey.

A WORLD-CLASS ATHLETE RUNS LIMBICALLY

Limbic walking and limbic running are not simply activities that the tribal people engaged in. All great athletes fall into it intuitively. Most practice it, in one form or another. This is how one great athlete puts it:

I don't want to know my time, because I don't want to discourage myself.

> John Campbell, age 41, Winner of the "Double Triple" (Los Angeles, Boston and New York City marathons 1989 and 1990), quoted in the August 1991 issue of *Runners World.*

John Campbell does not wear his watch when he runs. He tells us that he focuses on speed, but not on time. This is interesting because for most people speed has no meaning if not related to time. This is one succinct description of the limbic mode.

It seems to me that all great athletes are limbic during their peak experience. The spectators are cortical, largely because the commentators are cortical. It amuses me to listen to commentators and spectators attribute all types of "great intellectual strategies" to pitchers or batters. How many fractions of a second does a batter have after the ball leaves the pitcher's hand to think up a great intellectual strategy to hit the ball? In what state is a great pitcher as he faces a great batter? Is he intellectual about it — or is he limbic? In what state is a great tennis player when he serves to another great tennis player? How much time does the other player have to "read" the server, "analyze" the serve, "strategize" about it, adopt the "right" posture and then "cleverly" hit the ball? Likewise, how does a great basketball player do his thing on the court?

The demands of the cortical monkey are intense. At our games, we end up serving our cortical monkeys rather than savoring the game and feeling the limbic quality of the player's play.

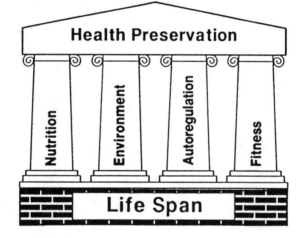

Chapter 3

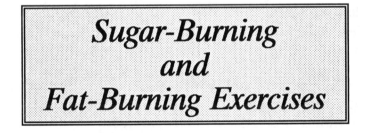

Limbic exercise combines physical exercise with meditation and self-regulation. The purpose is to achieve physical fitness of the body tissues and at the same time unclutter the mind. Of all the impediments to regular exercise, none is more insidious or unrelenting than a cluttered mind. From extensive personal experience with limbic exercise, and from the experience of my patients to whom I've recommended this method of exercise, I know that exercise done with an uncluttered mind is far more restorative than goal-oriented, competitive exercise. In my early work, it was not my intention to seek a deeper awareness of the essential spirituality of Man through limbic exercise. But this is indeed what happened not only to me but to several of my patients.

When in a limbic state, a person is free of all the usual thoughts that populate his mind. It is a native state of awareness of life, of energy and of a larger *presence* around us. It is a non-thinking but not a non-perceiving state. Limbic exercise means just that: exercising *limbically*. It does not mean that we plan our day while we exercise, nor that we review some past day during it.

The cortical monkey loves to recycle misery. When not content with recycling old miseries, it thrives on previewing the feared future miseries. In limbic exercise, we listen to our tissues; the energy of tissues banishes the cortical monkey. The energy of life makes irrelevant the things that happened but shouldn't have, or those that didn't happen but we wish had.

Clearly we all know exercise is essential for the fluidity of motion in our tissues. We know it is essential for long-term health. We are told it is required to keep our LDL cholesterol down, our HDL cholesterol high, our fat cells slim, our muscles firm and our cardiovascular status optimum. None of this, however, is relevant to limbic exercise. The core point is that in limbic exercise an awareness of energy and life and a larger presence around us replaces the usual quota of angry or sad thoughts, at least most of the time.

The cortical state drives humans to calculate, compute, compete and caution, and it creates images of disease and culminates in disease. The limbic condition, instead, cares, comforts, creates images of health and heals. In limbic exercise, it is not our purpose to achieve the health benefits of exercise by thinking more cleverly about its effects on our arteries, heart rhythm, brain waves or liver cell function. Rather, being limbic is to bring about physiologic changes *by a no-thinking approach.*

The principles and practice of autoregulation sometimes appear abstract to some of my patients, but this is usually a temporary problem. My book *The Cortical Monkey and Healing* discusses my concept of self-regulation and healing as it evolved during my work in clinical medicine over a period of about 30 years. In addition, I detail the critical differences between the limbic and cortical modes and explain how limbic listening is essential for self-regulation, while cortical clutter is a serious handicap. I recommend that book to the reader for valuable background information.

In developing an exercise program, I have adapted some methods of autoregulation for use with exercise. Before I discuss the subject of limbic exercise further, it is necessary for me to define the following terms:

1.   Cortical and Limbic Exercises
2.   Type I (slow twitch) and Type II (fast twitch)

Fibers
3.   Lipolytic and Glycolytic Exercises
4.   Energy, Fatigue and Stress Molecules
5.   Cortical and Limbic Pacing
6.   Cortical Greed and Limbic Gratitude
7.   Cortical Clutter and Limbic Openness
8.   Limbic Breathing

Cortical Exercises

Cortical exercises are intense, competitive, and goal-oriented. These exercises are of the *stop-and-go* type which focus on technique, style, duration and results. The best examples of cortical exercise are competition sports and athletics such as wrestling, bodybuilding, football, tennis, basketball and soccer. Sharply focused, highly intense and meticulously analyzed cortical exercises are evidently essential for such sports.

Limbic Exercises

Limbic exercises are *continuous,* non-intense, non-goal oriented, noncompetitive exercises. There is no hyperventilation or perspiration. When done *limbically*, exercise ends with more energy than that with which it began. The essence of limbic exercises is the *absence* of focus. When we run limbically, we do just that — we simply run. There is no effort made to run well, to run at some predetermined speed, to run for some defined distance or to run to solve the problems of the day. When we walk, we simply walk. We make no attempt to solve our problems or sit in judgment on how we walk. Limbic exercises are done with abandonment, with total disregard of all the demands of the thinking head.

Cortical exercises are performed while taking commands from the thinking mind. Limbic exercises, by contrast, are exercises done while we take counsel of our tissues, counsel from muscles that contract to produce motion, counsel from tendons that carry the commands from the muscles to the bones, counsel from the ligaments that hold the bones together and counsel from bones that provide muscles their scaffolds. We take counsel from lungs that bring air into the body and from the heart that pumps the blood to spread nourishment to the body tissues. A period of listening to body tissues (and dismissing all demands from the thinking mind — the cortical monkey) is a necessary prelude to limbic exercise. It generally requires several minutes before we begin limbic exercises. With continued limbic exercises comes what I call "limbic openness."

Limbic openness is a period of inner reflection, meditation, prayer and deep visceral stillness. There is no rush of cortical thoughts. There is only a *limbic* flow of limbic perceptions past one another. This subject is discussed at length later in this section.

Type I (slow twitch) Muscle Fibers

Type I muscle fibers burn fats to generate energy, much

like a candle burns wax to generate light slowly but for a long time. These muscle fibers are rich in mitochondria — and the oxidative enzymes contained in them. They are designed to break down fats and utilize the fatty acids liberated from fats by their oxidative enzymes.

Type II (fast twitch) Muscle Fibers

Type II muscle fibers burn sugar to generate quick bursts of energy, much like a piece of dry paper burns to produce sudden heat with a flash but only for a few moments. These muscle fibers have fewer mitochondria and are poor in mitochondrial oxidative enzymes. Unable to use fatty acids for energy, they follow the path of less resistance and burn whatever sugars are available to them (the glycolytic or sugar-burning molecular pathways for energy generation).

Lipolytic Exercises

Lipolytic exercises are fat-burning exercises. In these exercises, Type I muscle fibers *burn fat in a slow and sustained fashion*; the flame of the candle is subdued but it lasts for long periods of time. So it is that exercises that require a low but sustained supply of energy are predominantly lipolytic. Again, the myocyte (muscle cell) senses the energy needs and acts accordingly. In general, fat-burning exercises are limbic exercises.

Glycolytic Exercises

Glycolytic exercises are sugar-burning exercises. In these exercises, Type II muscle fibers burn sugars fast; the flame of the paper is bright but it dies out within moments. So it is that exercises that require rapid bursts of energy for short periods of time are predominantly sugar-burning. The myocyte *knows* it, is quick to sense the requirements for energy and acts accordingly. In general, sugar-burning exercises are cortical exercises.

Energy, Fatigue and Stress Molecules

One of the principal energy molecules in the human frame is ATP (adenosine triphosphate), while lactic acid is one of the principal fatigue molecules. Adrenaline and its cousin molecules catecholamines are the principal stress molecules. Although cortical exercises have many health advantages, when it comes to prolonging one's life span, the effects of cortical exercise are not as beneficial as those of limbic exercises. Cortical exercises *deplete* the body of its ATP energy molecules and increase the number of fatigue (lactic acid and others) and stress (adrenaline and others) molecules. Limbic exercise, by contrast, has the opposite effect: The number of lactic acid and adrenaline molecules is reduced and the number of ATP molecules is increased.

Cortical Pacing

Cortical pacing is the common method for determining the type, technique, speed and duration of exercise. This type of exercise pacing is highly goal-oriented, much like keeping a tight schedule at work. It includes the commonly used methods of "pushing the distance of the run," measuring the "pulse peak" and counting the breathing rate.

Limbic Pacing

Limbic pacing is a mode of exercise whereby a person allows himself to simply follow his inner "limbic voice." This voice may wish him to walk slowly or quickly, run with arms swinging from the shoulders or just hanging by the side; it may urge him to continue or stop.

Cortical Greed

Cortical greed is the irrepressible desire to "do autoregulation right." The core idea of autoregulation is to listen to the tissues by overcoming the unrelenting cortical demands for knowing what was, is and will be happening within our body tissues. These cortical demands negate the very idea of autoregulation. This is a point of enormous practical significance. Unquestionably, this has been the most common obstacle encountered by those patients of mine who have tried to learn autoregulation.

Limbic Gratitude

Limbic gratitude describes the sense of gratitude with which we accept whatever responses we receive from our tissues when we do autoregulation. Autoregulation, I reiterate, is about *listening to body tissues;* it is not putting demands on them. Limbic gratitude is gratitude in receiving, at a nonintellectual, limbic level.

Cortical Clutter

Cortical clutter is a term I use to convey the unending chatter in which we engage with our cortical minds. It is living in the head, an unremitting case of head fixation. It consists of all the What if, Why couldn't it, Why not, Why me and all of the other favorite lines we use for punishing our tissues. Unfortunately, canceling the cortical clutter is easier said than done.

There are other less threatening forms of cortical clutter, for example planning your day during your walk, or examining somebody else running on the same track, or simply not wanting to do exercises because it is Sunday or Saturday or the 4th of July. Most people who walk, run or cycle for fitness know what cortical clutter is, though the term may be unfamiliar to them: it is all the thoughts that cross their minds while exercising, all the problem-solving, head-clearing and goal-setting.

Anger and hostility are the first casualties of autoregulation. Walking or running without autoregulation is not nearly as effective in dissolving these serious threats to health and fitness as the same exercises when they are combined with autoregulation.

Limbic Openness

Golfers know what it is to be "on the greens." For tennis enthusiasts, it is being "on the courts" and for fishermen, "on the water." In autoregulation lingo, the term limbic openness describes a comforting limbic state in which there is no thought activity, no anger, no hostility, no desire to excel and no judgmental overview. It is a state of calm communion between what is under our skin with what is outside it. There is a consciousness of an openness, a wide, limitless, comforting limbic openness. In a more advanced state, there is a consciousness of a larger presence, a state totally free of any desire to map out, define, understand or know this presence. The presence is simply there.

I don't know if achieving the full depth and breadth of limbic openness is possible for most people during limbic exercise. Perhaps not. What I know from both personal experience and that of some of my patients is that limbic openness in some form or other is attainable by most people through limbic exercise. At the very least, most people who practice limbic exercise learn to allow themselves an escape from cortical clutter without much difficulty. For many individuals, it may indeed require considerable practice.

Limbic Breathing

Limbic breathing is a specific type of breathing that significantly lowers the blood level of lactic acid, adrenaline and other catecholamines. There is strong but indirect evidence that limbic exercises also prevent depletion of ATP energy molecules. I describe in detail the specifics of this type of breathing in *The Cortical Monkey and Healing,* of which excerpts appear at the end of this chapter.

Extensive experience with autoregulation and other non-drug treatment protocols for the reversal of immune and degenerative disorders has convinced me of the central place of limbic breathing in the healing process. That work — and my conviction based upon it — raised the possibility that limbic breathing might be of great value in limbic exercise. This indeed did happen soon after I started experiments with such breathing during my own daily exercises.

WHY DON'T MOST PEOPLE EXERCISE?

The most common answers to this question are:
I should but ....
I don't have the energy.
Flogging of will and commitment.
I don't have the time.
I walk fast.
I walk a lot at work.
I hate it. It is the most boring thing.
My legs become sore.
Can only do one big activity a day. I can do my shopping or I can exercise.
Where can I go to exercise?
I don't need to run *away* from anything.

Something always hurts me.

I would do it if I could do it all my life. But I know I cannot do that.

The extra few months that I might live by doing exercise every day are not worth it.

Most people can relate to one or more of the preceding responses. All of them are based on the assumption that physical exercise, of necessity, is an unpleasant intrusion on one's life. This, of course, is the crux of the matter in our present discussion of limbic exercise. For exercise to be a part of one's day, it must come to us naturally and effortlessly. It should be free of any requirements of "planning." Exercise to increase one's life span must have an element of spontaneity to it. Just as we spontaneously do many things during the day without any preparation or premeditation, we should be able to do the same with exercise. I quote here the words of John Casti, a mathematician of some renown.

> "*That way, perhaps, those of us destined for middle-aged spread could be genetically altered to remain eternally slim and trim without the need to devote hours of valuable sleeping, eating, and drinking time to things like jogging, pumping iron, and quaffing bottles of those ghastly diet sodas.*"

John Casti, of course, wrote those words in jest (I think). But the notion of exercise as a waste of valuable sleeping, eating and drinking time is widespread. The real reason for this is not that the cortical monkey does not see the value in physical fitness. Nor that he really does not understand the hollowness of these statements. Nor that the issue in limbic exercise is not that we are merely scheming to live a few months longer. Not that we are looking for the endorphin high. The cortical monkey knows all this only too well.

What time can be more treasured than deeply personal time without any agendas? The cortical monkey knows this. What can be more cherished than reaching, and staying, in limbic openness? A state in which there is no thought activity, no judgment, no right, no wrong, no past hurts, no present misery, no feared future suffering? This is also well known to the cortical monkey. The real problem is that the cortical monkey cannot help himself. He is destined to struggle relentlessly to suppress limbic openness. It is the nature of the beast. He fights limbic openness tooth and nail. Why? Because he cannot exist there.

We can find time for exercise,
or we can save time for illness.

MOTIVATION FOR LIMBIC EXERCISE

The subject of motivation fascinates me, and I find motivation "experts" to be fascinating people. Consider the following quote:

> *The purpose of this article is to examine movement science research on personal and social-environmental motivational influence in physical activity contexts. Motivation is defined as a process in which internal and external factors direct and energize thoughts, feelings, and actions. Motivation is described as a consequence of meaning, which is derived from a combination of personal and social factors, including personal goals or incentives, expectations of personal efficiency, movement-related perceptual and affective experience, and social and physical features of the environment.*

> *Physical Therapy* 70:808; 1990

When I read the above lines I squirmed. The language of this motivational piece intimidated me as I imagine they would almost anyone. I read the piece a second time. No relief. A time to escape, I told myself. I went limbic.

I wonder how many people will read such an article and become so motivated that they will jump up and run out for some exercise. The subject of exercise is not pleasant for many of us. It conjures up images of boredom (endless running), lost time (too busy to exercise) and sore legs. Running on the street, missing the step on the curb and spraining an ankle. How often do street runners wear those awful, tortured looks? Stooping down, ready to collapse. Inhaling air rich in diesel exhaust. Who ordered this punishment? Self-flagellation? What are they running from anyway? *Movement-related perceptual and affective experiences?* No thanks, you say. Go ahead, call me a couch potato. At least I like what I do.

If exercise is to successfully reverse catabolic maladaptation, it must first be good enough to be desired. Not only at an intellectual level, but at a deeper limbic level. If the butterfly is to find its escape, it must first recognize the illusion of the skylight glass. This is the essence of limbic exercise.

YOU WANT TO COME OUT — BUT YOU DON'T WANT TO COME OUT

People who learn autoregulation know well what the above statement means. So do those who meditate regularly. As a person goes deep into autoregulation, escaping into limbic openness, he wants to stay there. But most of us know we cannot stay there forever. There is the day's work waiting for us. So it is that when most of the time I do autoregulation myself (including when I teach it to my patients), I want to come out of it, but I don't want to come out of it. This phenomenon is real. Auto-reggers know it. Meditators know it. People who pray know it.

The principle of limbic exercise took shape in my mind

during one of my limbic exercise periods. After initial muscle stretching and some rope jumping, I started doing my rug-running (which as I indicated earlier is running in place on a three feet by three feet piece of rug). Within minutes I fell into the limbic rhythm of running and passed into limbic openness. Sometime later I came around and wondered how long I had been doing my limbic run. My first urge was to stop for a moment and check the time. My next urge was to keep going for a little while, just as it had happened to me on innumerable occasions during my autoregulation periods. I wanted to come out of limbic running, and I didn't want to come out. So here was a solution to the problem of boredom in exercise: Go limbic during exercise and dissipate all sense of boredom. These urges of wanting to get out and yet not wanting to get out were to become a regular part of my limbic exercise until I became convinced that this phenomenon was real. Further validation of this phenomenon came to me (as it did in my other observations of autoregulation) through some of my patients.

THE BATTLE OF A SPLIT SECOND

Most of us know this battle. We win or lose with this battle. It is the battle between the cortical monkey and us every time we have to do something that we know is good and necessary. Sometimes it takes the form of turning down that second cup of coffee or better still, that first cup. At other times, it is the moment when we make a good food choice over a poor one. And, of course, it is *the* battle when it comes to limbic exercise. The cortical monkey is an inventive animal. It comes up with a million reasons why exercise may be delayed today or perhaps even postponed till tomorrow. It never fails for the beginner. For him, it is a killer. For the veteran, the monkey's pranks are but a matter of some amusement.

There is only one way of winning this battle: Don't engage the cortical monkey.

SAHIB, SOCHO MUTT

"Sahib, socho mutt." This was the advice an old foot soldier gave to his young major many years ago. Not bad advice for going limbic.

During a recent trip to Newport, Rhode Island, my brother-in-law, Major Ilyas Khan, and I were walking on the beach. He was very interested in my research methods of limbic exercise. At one point he recalled a piece of advice one of his foot soldiers gave him during a "forced march." In the infantry, a forced march, he told me, is a very long march with heavy, full gear on the backs of soldiers. On one occasion, the march was to be over fifty miles long and to take the soldiers along dirt roads through hilly countryside. Understandably, the young soldiers were preoccupied with the length of the march and with the sore legs and blistered feet with which they expected to return. The major didn't quite know how to reassure his command. The old foot soldier sensed his plight.

"Sahib, socho mutt," the foot soldier told his major.

The urdu word socho means thinking. Mutt means don't. Sahib stands for sir. Sir, don't think. Simply walk. That is what the foot soldier really meant. Going limbic is as old as human experience. It takes different forms in different times and in different cultures. The words change, the essence of being limbic does not. The words of the foot soldier could easily have been, "Sir, don't engage the cortical monkey. He does not let up just because we choose to exercise. He loves to debate. And you cannot win."

A THOUGHT STOPS ME IN MID-STEP

Most people who walk or run know how bad thoughts stop them in mid-step. It happens to all of us. Most of us do not fully appreciate this phenomenon unless we become aware of it.

The cortical monkey is a tenacious creature. It is a clever inventor of excuses. Just as this monkey springs many traps for us when we are not exercising, it does so while we exercise. Some cortical impulses are literally paralyzing. The "thought" (the battle of split seconds), in essence, is a cortical trap set up by the cortical monkey. Professional athletes devise special strategies for dealing with this phenomenon. People who run for their health frequently fall prey to the mischief of the cortical monkey. Some favorite phrases of the cortical monkey sound like this:

It is Saturday today.
It might rain today.
Today, I am not up to it.
I walk with Sally. She is not walking today.
Do I have to do this every day? That new study showed
exercise done on alternate days is good enough.
I did exercise yesterday.
I should have been on vacation by now.
I stayed on my diet yesterday.

And so on.

THE BATTLE OF MINUTES

After the beginner wins the battle of the split second with the cortical monkey, he faces the second battle of the minutes. This is the battle with cortical messages he receives from his leg muscles, usually within minutes of starting limbic exercises. The legs become sore and the feet heavy. The cortical message is simple: Stop this unwanted work. Sometimes the cortical messages are terse: Put an end to this misery. The beginner needs a strategy for this battle. Changing the type and speed of exercise is a reliable weapon in this battle. I discuss this subject further later in this volume.

Another good strategy is that of "sarkari double."

SARKARI DOUBLE

There is another expression common in the Pakistani military. The soldiers learn to run limbically when they would rather not run at all. They call it "sarkari double." This is in reality limbic running into which they intuitively fall. In this running, they do not follow any external signals or cues. They have no goals. When they run, they simply run. They are unburdened by any cortical commands.

MORE ON
CORTICAL GREED AND LIMBIC GRATITUDE

We Americans are a numerical people. We Americans, it seems to me, must live by numbers. Numbers must define the "amount" of joy we *must* extract from our lives. Numbers must determine how long we walk. Numbers must define how fast we walk. The pulse-count numbers must tell us when to speed up. The breathing-rate count must tell us when to slow down. Numbers must define the thickness of the soles of our walking shoes. And the number of days we must walk. And the number of times we must talk to whomever will listen to us about the number of days we walk.

Counting is "cortical greed." When we celebrate our famous pulse count or the breathing rate, little do we realize that the process of counting increases the pulse and makes the breathing a little bit heavier, a little bit more labored. I know, because I study almost every single one of my patients electrophysiologically to assess how their cortical monkeys punish their body tissues.

SHORT VERSUS LONG BOUTS OF EXERCISE

There is an active debate among the exercise experts as to how many minutes one should exercise to get the most benefit. Alas, the numbers again! Why is it that we Americans must ruin the fun in everything by putting some numbers on it?

A regimen of moderately intense exercise for periods of 30 minutes three times per week is very popular with many researchers studying methods for increasing exercise training and functional capacity. Indeed, the 30-minute duration seems to have assumed divine rights among our exercise experts.

The exercise gurus at the American Heart Association have pronounced that we can get some physical benefits out of exercise only if we do it for a minimum of 30 minutes. These gurus also prescribe methods of exercise that will give us a pulse count of which they approve; the target heart rate, they advise, should "represent 70 percent of the maximum treadmill rate".

What happened to common sense? Why has it become so uncommon? A victim of our numbers?

Thus, multiple short bouts of moderate-intensity exercise training significantly increase peak oxygen uptake. For many individuals short bouts of exercise training may fit better into a busy schedule than a single long bout.

Am J Cardiol 65:1010; 1990

So a new band of young Turks are defying the *high priests* of the American Heart Association. Where will it all end?

The authors of the above report write,

To evaluate the "threshold" of exercise duration required to produce training effects we compared ....

So what do we do when we simply feel a desire to walk or run or swim or bicycle? Wonder about the "threshold" of exercise duration required to produce the "training effects"?

They continue,

The solid state recorder enabled accurate quantitation of the exercise regimen for both groups.

Numbers again! When simply counting the pulse is not enough, we wire ourselves with solid state recorders. How many "busy executives" whom these investigators wish to help in their exercise program will now begin to carry solid state recorders? How many of them will be obsessed with what the recorder is recording while they run? How many of them will tighten their arteries wondering about the "threshold" of exercise required by them to produce "training effects"? So much for cortical greed.

FUNNIES IN MEDICINE

I read medical literature as a hobby. It has its light moments. I have often wondered why medical writings are called medical "literature." Literature is the search for truth. Literature is about the human condition. Literature is about the reach of imagination. And imagination is not what we physicians write about. Indeed, *imagining* about things is taboo in modern medicine. Yes, there is an element of search in medical writings today. But it is about the search for new drugs, or at least about new ways of prescribing old drugs. It is almost never about the human condition.

Quite apart from their literary quality, medical writings often carry unintended but rewarding bits of humor. Consider the following quotes:

"Listen to your body" is a phrase patients often recall after a visit to a physician.

New Jersey Medicine 88:658; 1991

"Great! I like it." I spoke out loud when I read it first. This is good stuff. Listening to the body. This is what this book is all about. Then it occurred to me I had read something about drugs in the preceding pages. I turned the page and found the lines I was looking for (page 657).

Patients who do not routinely take NSAIDs often will benefit from pretreatment with these drugs prior to their exercise.

NSAIDs (nonsteroidal anti-inflammatory drugs), of course, are drugs that are used for arthritis, and that regularly cause stomach erosions, often leading to gastritis and bleeding. What amused me most was the writer's advice to people with arthritis that they should take drugs even if they "do not routinely take NSAIDs."

Listening to Drugs?

I must admit this was my first exposure to the implicit concept of listening to drugs. Clearly, if we listen to our bodies after we drug ourselves, we will listen to the drugs and not to our bodies. *We physicians love our drugs, don't we*? On the rare occasions when we do advise our patients to listen to their bodies, we ask them first to load themselves up with drugs.

THE EXPLORER

There was an explorer in all of us at one time. That explorer was inquisitive, inventive and always eager to experiment. He looked at life the way it came to him, taking one moment at a time. He had energy, fluidity of mind and was willing to try things out. The explorer didn't much care for all the things that go wrong. He just did things, without analysis, without critique, without goals.

Most of us lose that explorer along the way, a victim of the unrelenting demands of the cortical monkey. Cortical clutter suffocates this explorer. We need to find that explorer and bring him back. For limbic exercises, we need his spontaneity, his willingness, his way of looking at life. We need this explorer back with us for limbic exercises.

Medical education sometimes seems to me designed to destroy the explorer in us. Medical students are ingenious young men when they enter medical schools. But then their thinking is sanitized. They arrive at our medical offices and the hospital wards as "trained physicians," their brains teeming with statistics, cleansed of all holistic notions about health, and cluttered with the names of rare syndromes that they will seldom, if ever, encounter among their real patients. The explorer dies, except when he tinkers with drugs or medical gadgets of Star Wars Medicine.

LIMBIC LIPOLYTIC
AND CORTICAL GLYCOLYTIC EXERCISES

Energy in foods exists as a chemical bond energy. Living bodies require electromagnetic, thermal (heat) and mechanical forms of energy. The purpose of metabolism is to convert the chemical bond energy of foods to those other forms of energy for the performance of various life functions.

In the catabolic maladaptation of obesity, the primary dysfunction is that of energy generation. The enzymes essential for energy are either very sluggish due to disuse and loss of muscle mass, or are poisoned by denatured and toxic foods, pesticides and herbicides, environmental pollution, allergic reactions, oxidizing molecules of stress and various forms of radiation. All these factors lead to the collection of excess fat and toxic fatty substances in the fat cells.

How can we reverse this catabolic maladaptation? In *The Butterfly and Life Span Nutrition,* I describe strategies for preventing enzyme inactivation and toxicity with food choices. In this section, I will discuss how we can replenish the fat-burning enzymes in the muscle fibers. To do so, first I need to cover certain essential aspects of muscle physiology.

SUGAR-BURNING EXERCISES
VERSUS
FAT-BURNING EXERCISES

When a bodybuilder exercises, he does so to build his muscles. For this purpose, by and large, he needs short bursts of high-energy output. The muscle cells that respond are primarily of the Type II (fast twitch) myocytes, which predominantly burn sugars to produce quick bursts of energy. These myocytes are poor in fat-burning mitochondrial oxidative enzymes. The very nature of exercise undertaken by the body-builder puts him into a sugar-burning catabolic mode. The bodybuilders know how quickly they lose muscle mass and become flabby and obese when they stop their bodybuilding exercises.

When a marathon runner runs, the muscle fibers that primarily respond to his activity are of Type I (slow twitch) myocytes, which are rich in fat-burning oxidative mitochondrial enzymes. These enzymes burn fat at a slow and sustained rate, very much like a candle does, slowly and for long periods of time.

If an overweight person says he loves his exercise time, he is probably being polite. His fat-burning enzymes are sluggish (often totally exhausted). He is not likely to find much pleasure in beating up on the tired enzymes and tired tissues. If a slim, energetic person says the same thing, the chances are he means it. His enzymes are charged, his tissues energized.

The problems of the bodybuilder when he stops exercising and of the overweight person *are not problems of the mind.* These are problems of sluggish enzymes and neglected Type I myocytes. The advantages of the runner and those of the slim, energetic person *are also not advantages of the mind.* These are physiologic advantages of charged enzymes and pampered Type I myocytes.

Chapter 4

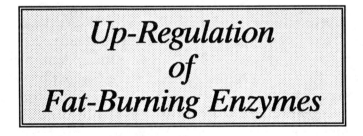

Health is harmony among cells. Harmony among cells is synergy among their enzymes. What are enzymes?

ENZYMES ARE WHAT SEPARATE
LIVING ORGANISMS FROM NONLIVING OBJECTS

Enzymes are molecules that give living things the *quality* of life. Enzymes are catalysts in biologic reactions; these molecules facilitate reactions among other molecules but, in general, are not used up in those reactions. They make things happen. Indeed, enzymes *are* life.

There are two fundamental defects of enzyme function in the United States today: 1) The fat-burning enzymes are down-regulated; and 2) The sugar-burning enzymes are dysregulated. The fat-burning enzymes are clogged by oxidized and denatured fats in the standard American diet. The sugar-burning enzymes are overdriven by the enormous sugar overload in our diet. I include below some brief comments about what enzymes are and how they function in molecular metabolic and defense pathways.

Man has not been able to fully understand what life is. His science has not been able to define what life is. Since the time modern man walked out of the Rift Valley in Central Africa (or so paleohistorians want us to believe), he has searched for the true meaning of life and has failed consistently.

In frustration, he has expressed the essential nature of life as *vital force, life force, energy force* or simply *vitality*. Indeed, the poet and the philosopher have always been closer to describing the *quality* of life than the scientist.

ENZYMES: THE LIFE FORCE IN NATURE

To understand what enzymes are and how they function, let us consider the example of automobile wheels moving on a road surface. When the road surface is dry, the wheels hug the road and the driver is in easy command of his vehicle. When it rains and the road surface is wet, the wheels do not hug the road as well. The driver senses this change and slows down to improve his control over his vehicle. During a freezing rain, ice prevents the wheels from hugging the road surface, and the vehicle slides uncontrollably. If the driver does not slow his vehicle to a crawl or a stop, he may find himself in a ditch by the roadside. How does this happen? The answer: The water reduces the friction between the tire and the road (facilitates the interaction between the two). The play of the tire on the road surface is looser and freer, and it loses its grip on the road surface. The driver senses some difficulty of control. When water freezes, the smooth surface of the ice almost completely eliminates friction between the tire and the road surface. The driver cannot cope with such rapid play of the tire on the road unless he slows down.

In the above analogy, water acts as an enzyme. It is not used up but simply facilitates the movement (interaction) between the surfaces of the tire and the road (reduces friction between the two in common language). So enzymes are life molecules that *make things happen in living organisms.*

The subject of exercise cannot be dissociated from the subject of foods. Foods in nature are living things. Enzymes are what give foods in nature their life. Indeed, enzymes *are* the life in foods. If this is true, why is the subject of enzymes in human nutrition almost completely neglected by our nutrition experts? The answer to this question has something to do with the limitations of the available methods of scientific inquiry. The prevailing research models do not allow us to fully understand the *quality* of life in enzymes.

It is essential to recognize that what brings proteins, fats, carbohydrates and minerals to life is enzymes. Without enzymes, these substances would be nothing but lifeless masses of molecules. Casimer Funk recognized the *vital* importance of some substances to health, and his "substances" were called *vitamins.* Most vitamins *are* enzymes. Those that do not meet the biochemical characteristics to be considered enzymes primarily act to facilitate enzymes.

MOLECULAR PUNISHMENT BY NIGHT

I often hear people planning to exercise in order to "burn

off" their excess fat. This is an illusion of biology.

Let us consider what happens when two friends go out for dinner in the evening. They have a couple of drinks and follow it up with a large meal of rolls with butter, rich creamy soup, thick steak, potato with sour cream, and a layered chocolate cake for dessert. They have a couple of more drinks before retiring for sleep. One of the friends is slim and lean while the other is 35% over his optimal life span weight. How does metabolism deal with such a meal in the absence of catabolic maladaptation (in the lean person)? How does it respond to this load in the presence of catabolic maladaptation (in the obese person)?

A heavy dinner like the one described above may add up to over 2,000 calories. On a purely numerical basis, a pound of fat stores about 3,500 calories. An average person will need to walk over seven miles to burn off this many calories. But rather than walk over seven miles, both individuals in this situation go to sleep.

THE ENZYME FURNACE

Each living cell has an enzyme furnace. Food fuels this furnace; exercise stokes its fire. This furnace self-regulates. It adjusts its rate of combustion in response to the demands put upon it. The efficiency of this furnace determines whether the food melts away in our tissues or it "sticks" to them.

The slim friend has vigorous, up-regulated fat-burning enzymes that expediently break down his meal and use up the energy in calories during his sleep. His enzyme furnace is stoked well even as he sleeps. His enzymes work feverishly to metabolize his dinner and spare his fat cells the extra caloric load. The fat-burning enzymes in the overweight friend, by contrast, are down-regulated, sluggish, or worse, exhausted. There is little fire left in his enzyme furnace. He suffers molecular punishment by night without even knowing it. His fat cells suffocate with yet more fat as he sleeps.

The core point in our discussion is this: The purpose of limbic exercise is to keep the fat-burning mitochondrial enzymes up-regulated and in an optimal functional state. The key issue is the rate of enzymatic activity. It is not to burn off calories.

Down-regulation of fat-burning enzymes is the basic derangement of the catabolic maladaptation that I discussed at length in the companion volume *The Butterfly and Life Span Nutrition*. When catabolic maladaptation does not exist, the calories contained in big meals are rapidly used up. When the catabolic maladaptation does exist, the calories in the meal are stored as excess fat in the fat cells, causing further deterioration in the catabolic status and adding to the problem of obesity.

"Dr. Ali, food sticks to me. My doctor thinks I have a fertile imagination."

A patient once spoke these words in frustration. He had failed to lose weight with several dieting attempts. It is not uncommon for me to hear people talk about how the "food sticks" to some individuals and simply melts away in others. The molecular equivalent of food sticking to some bodies, of course, is down-regulated enzymes. This is the molecular and energy basis of this common observation. How do we physicians, incarcerated in our drug medicine as we are, look at this issue? During all my years in medical school, residency training and clinical practice, not once did I receive any education about how down-regulated enzymes cause obesity. I did, however, hear an awful lot of my colleagues deride their patients for such simple-minded thinking. As a physician colleague put it once, the common form of obesity is a glandular problem only if you consider the mouth as a gland.

HOW SAD IS SAD?

The standard American diet (SAD) is a sad affair of oxidized, denatured and depleted foods. How toxic is the oil heated to 200° to 300° that our fast food outlets use to cook French fries for our children? These oils are cesspools of oxidized fats, trans fatty acids and toxic cyclic peroxides. How salty are our snacks? How sugary are our drinks? How healthy are our meats taken from cattle fed steroids for growth? And our fish taken from fisheries sprinkled with fungicides? How do these toxic molecules poison our fat-burning enzymes? How toxic is American food? How sad is SAD? These questions cannot be answered without a basic understanding of the essential chemistry of life. I discuss the essentials of the basic chemistry of life for general readers without any chemistry background at length in the companion volume *The Butterfly and Life Span Nutrition.* I reproduce below some text from that book as a frame of reference for discussing how fat-burning enzymes are down-regulated and how they can be up-regulated.

NATURE HAS ITS OWN ECONOMY

Nature has its own designs for its economy. Nature is not wasteful. Recycling life is Nature's master stroke.

Each living thing must one day die. If it had not been so for one single life form, that life form would have lived forever and would have crowded out all other forms of life from the planet Earth.

If one species of fish had lived forever, it would have filled up all the oceans, seas, rivers and lakes on our planet. There would have been no room for any other species of fish. Or for any other form of life in the water, any mollusk, any crab, any algae. If one single species of plant or animal on earth were to be exempt from nature's "law of death", that plant or animal would have packed every inch of the land. There would have been no room for a new twig, a new bloom, a new plant, a new insect or a new baby. I wonder if Gilgamesh knew this.

How did nature design this death-life-death cycle? Nature is master planner. It is an ingenious designer. It has its own economy. It rarely errs. It is self-correcting.

Oxidation is nature's grand design for assuring that no life form lives forever. Nature made oxidation a spontaneous process. It requires no expenditure of energy. It needs no external cues or outside programming. In scientific jargon, oxidation is defined as *loss* of electrons by atoms and molecules. A molecule is a group of atoms bonded together. Electrons are the tiniest packets of energy. When atoms and molecules lose electrons, they lose energy. In oxidation, high-energy atoms and molecules are changed into lower-energy level atoms and molecules. *This is the essence of the phenomenon of aging.*

In the mid-sixties, Bjorksten and Harmon put forth their theories of protein cross-linking and free radical injury respectively as the basic mechanisms of the aging process. Healthy threadlike protein molecules normally occur in different sizes. Individual molecules are bent and turned and twisted into many different shapes. Yet, they fight hard to preserve their individuality. The term cross-linking means these molecules are torn apart and when the ends unite, they get tangled with each other and form crooked protein molecules. Cross-linked molecules are two molecules wrapped around each other in such a way that neither can function normally. What molecular events cause protein cross-linking? Oxidative injury. It is the oxidant molecules that tear apart the healthy protein molecules and lead to tangling and cross-linking of these molecules.

How does free radical injury begin? What are free radicals? Free radical injury begins with oxidative injury. Free radicals are highly unstable, extremely reactive atoms or molecules that form when oxidant molecules injure other molecules. Aging of human tissues and molecules cannot take place by free radical injury unless these radicals are first produced as a result of oxidation. It follows that *spontaneity of oxidation* in human tissues, and oxidative molecular injury that results, may be regarded as the *true* nature of the aging process in man. Tissue capacity for anti-oxidant generation (production of life span molecules to control the aging-oxidant molecules and related molecules called oxyradicals) is determined by certain genetic and acquired factors. Life span molecules so produced provide the essential molecular counterbalance to spontaneous oxidation. I draw the evidence for this viewpoint from a large body of clinical and experimental data.

THE AGING-OXIDANT MOLECULES (AOMs)

During the early period of the development of my theory of aging-oxidant and life span foods, I often wondered if these two descriptions adequately conveyed my ideas of health and fitness to my patients. I started using these terms tentatively in my seminars on nutrition for the life span. I soon discovered that patients without any biology background at all could understand them, and the essential ideas behind their use easily and effortlessly. Indeed, people found the simplified concept of molecular aging, disease and death described with these two terms a useful framework for understanding nutrition. Below is a brief explanation of these terms.

The AOMs exist to assure that no life form lives forever. These molecules are present in each flower, each plant, each animal and each person. These are powerful molecules, fully capable of instantaneously burning all tissues. The AOMs can be divided into two broad categories: the internal metabolic AOMs and the external synthetic and natural toxic AOMS. The examples of the first category include aging-oxidant metabolic enzymes, minerals, proteins, fats and stress molecules. The external AOMs include industrial pollutants, petrochemicals, synthetic household chemicals, antibiotics, pesticides and herbicides. Radioactivity, ultraviolet waves and other forms of radiation do not come under the strict definition of AOMs, but readily generate AOMs by acting upon various atoms and molecules.

THE LIFE SPAN MOLECULES (LSMs)

Life span molecules are molecules that provide a counterbalance to aging-oxidant molecules. These molecules exist to assure that the aging-oxidant molecules do not cause instant combustion of all living forms. As each flower, each plant, each animal and each person is made up of AOMs, so it is made up of LSMs. LSMs exist to provide a counterbalance to AOMs. These molecules "neutralize" AOMs and prevent unwanted tissue damage. It is their responsibility to assure that each life form gets the opportunity to live out its normal life span in health, and with vigor and vitality. Examples of such molecules are vitamins, essential fatty acids, essential amino acids, essential minerals, and other antioxidants.

THE LIFE SPAN AND AGING-OXIDANT ENZYMES

Historically, the enzymes in the human body have been classified into two broad groups: the digestive enzymes and the metabolic enzymes. This was a valid classification. I say it *was* because this classification was developed and taught before we realized the devastating impact of synthetic chemicals and toxic metals on human biology.

From an ecologic viewpoint, it seems to me, it is useful to separate enzymes into *life span enzymes* (enzymes that support life span molecules) and *aging-oxidant enzymes* (enzymes that facilitate the destructive-oxidative function of aging-oxidant molecules). Just as nature designed some molecules to assure that no life form lives forever, it designed some enzymes for the same reason. Similarly, life span enzymes were designed to sustain the living organisms for their life span.

The enzymes in our model of aging-oxidant and life span molecules can be divided into two broad categories: 1) Aging-oxidant enzymes that support the aging-oxidant molecules and make sure no living organism lives forever; and 2) Life span enzymes that counterbalance the aging-oxidant enzymes and assure that living organisms do get an opportunity to live out their expected life spans.

What are the clinical implications of this viewpoint of aging in man? Oxygen is a molecular Dr. Jekyll and Mr. Hyde. Life-sustaining aspects of oxygen are well understood in clinical medicine. Life-terminating capability of oxygen is generally ignored. Man today faces extinction by accelerated oxidative molecular damage much like proto-eukaryotes did during an earlier era. This accelerated oxidative stress is caused by the impact upon his genetic makeup of an enormous overload of aging-oxidant molecules on his internal and external environment. What are the best strategies for health promotion and reversal of chronic immunologic and degenerative disorders? These are the strategies that address *all* aspects of accelerated oxidative molecular injury. These are the clinical management protocols of nutritional medicine, environmental medicine, medicine of self-regulation and medicine of fitness. Integrated applications of such management protocols define the clinical practice of molecular medicine.

What is the language of molecular injury?

Oxidation.

****

What is the language of molecular recovery?

Reduction.

****

What is the language of molecular aging?

Oxidative molecular injury.

****

What is the true nature of the aging process?

Spontaneity of oxidation in nature.

Buzz words are central to the American experience. Aerobics is the great buzz word of the gurus of fitness of our time. There is hardly an aspect of physical activity that fascinates us more than the subjects of aerobic and anaerobic exercises.

Max VO₂, AEROBIC AND ANAEROBIC EXERCISES

The terms aerobic and anaerobic mean "with oxygen" and "without oxygen" respectively. Aerobic metabolism is tissue metabolism with sufficient oxygen to break down food and body stores of fats, carbohydrates and proteins completely to yield energy. The anaerobic metabolism, by contrast, is a type of metabolism in which complete breakdown of food or body stores cannot take place due to an inadequate supply of oxygen. During anaerobic metabolism, lactic acid and other fatigue molecules accumulate in the tissues and call to a halt all physical activity.

The term Max VO_2 refers to the maximum amount of oxygen which the body can utilize at any given time. Exercise physiologists use this term for maximal aerobic capacity. Increase your Max VO_2 and you will improve your performance — so goes the conventional advice from exercise experts. Translation: Do speed work to push the cardiovascular and respiratory systems and improve the function of Type II muscle fibers. To support this advice with scientific studies, these exercise experts cite Swedish studies involving experienced distance runners. The results showed that runners who did speed work increased the efficiency of their Type II fibers more than those who ran twice as much but did so aerobically. Such studies clearly are of great value to those in competition distance running, but are of little concern to us.

Is Max VO$_2$ of great significance for us in our discussion of limbic exercise? The plain answer: little, if any. We are not interested in improving the form and function of Type II "fast twitch" muscle cells in our legs. These are sugar-burning cells. For ideal health and life span weight we want to increase the efficiency of fat-burning "slow twitch" muscle fibers *in all parts of the body.*

UP-REGULATION OF FAT-BURNING ENZYMES WITH LIMBIC EXERCISE

How are fat-burning enzymes down-regulated? I wrote earlier that our fat-burning enzymes are injured by denatured, oxidized fats in our food, by environmental pollutants, and by lack of slow, sustained exercise that enhances the form and function of these enzymes. It follows that successful strategies for up-regulation of these enzymes must address these same issues. I discuss nutritional requirements for this purpose in *The Butterfly and Life Span Nutrition.* I discuss some essential aspects of the environmental pollutants on human biology in *The Canary and Chronic Fatigue.* In this chapter, I discuss some essential aspects of up-regulation of fat-burning enzymes and normalization of sugar-burning enzymes with exercise.

LITTLE ANTHONY AND MOM'S ENZYMES

Little Anthony wandered around between the aisles of a supermarket. His mom ambled beside her toddler son, picking up a can of one food here and a bottle of another there. The inner workings of her muscles were the farthest thing from her mind. Minutes later, she paid at the checkout counter and walked out, little Anthony still by her side. Outside in the parking lot, little Anthony suddenly dashed after a piece of a colorful gift wrap blown by the wind. His mom saw a fast-moving car approach her toddler son from the corner of her one eye. She froze on her feet, paralyzed with fear, her throat choking in terror. Then she lunged forward in a frenzy and snapped him out of the way of the car.

How did the muscles in her legs know they needed to produce energy at a slow, even rate when she walked in comfort between the aisles of the supermarket? How did they know they needed to produce quick bursts of energy out in the parking lot? People in the mind-over-body business concoct elegant theories to explain how all this happens. I do not know much about those theories. To me it is simply a matter of enzymes doing what they were designed to do. It is a matter of intelligence of energy enzymes in the muscle fibers.

One can argue that the voluntary muscles are under our

voluntary control. It still doesn't solve our problem. Muscle cells get their orders from the mind. Where do the enzymes get their orders?

How do enzymes know all this? It seems safe to say that 50 years from now — or perhaps in 20 years — our understanding of how enzymes work will be much greater than at present. Will we then understand the intelligence and will of enzymes?

ENZYMES KNOW

I do not know if man will ever fully know the intelligence of energy enzymes. Still, while such goals might forever elude us, there is enough known about the structure and function of enzymes for us to dispel several popular but frivolous notions about exercise, weight loss and human life span.

Insights into the workings of muscle cells can come only through an understanding of these phenomena. The energy and molecular events that occur in muscle cells are easy to understand for everyone. A biology background is neither necessary for an understanding of these phenomena nor is it required to learn how disturbances in these mechanisms can cause dis-ease and eventually lead to disease.

The muscles in Anthony's mom have two main types of muscle cells: Type I red, slow-twitch muscle cells and Type II white, fast-twitch muscle cells. The Type I muscle cells are rich in oxidative, fat-burning enzymes. These cells produce energy in a slow, sustained fashion, predominantly by burning fat in an aerobic state — when oxygen is freely available for this purpose. Type I fibers have low ATPase enzyme activity. When a thin section of the muscle is strained for this enzyme, it takes a minimal quantity of the enzyme stain and appears very pale when examined with a microscope. (My editor crossed out "with" in the preceding sentence and inserted "under" in its place. I have actually tried to examine things by placing them *under* the microscope. The bases of microscopes are usually made up of metals and nothing can be examined by putting it *under* the microscope.) Mom's Type I generated just enough energy for her to comfortably walk beside her toddler between the supermarket aisles. When she stopped to look at some labels or pick some items, these muscle cells produced just enough energy to let her stand up against the pull of gravity and maintain her posture.

The leg muscles of Anthony's mom also contain Type II white, fast-twitch cells. These cells are rich in sugar-burning enzymes, and well-designed for quick-fire energy required for intense activities for short periods of time. With ATPase stain, these muscle cells stain dark, indicating the high quantity and activity of this enzyme in them. Out in the parking lot, these muscles came into play to carry her legs as she leaped to pull her toddler back from the speeding car.

The mom in our story was a lithesome, athletic young woman who ran for fitness. During her pregnancy, she rapidly gained weight and experienced progressive fatigue. Exercise of even a moderate degree became difficult for her. Several months later, she joined a gym. Within weeks, she lost weight, gained back her lost stamina, and felt energetic and free of fatigue. How did this all happen?

Nature has its own economy. It abhors waste. Nature, it seems to me, has two main strategies for its economy: recycling and diversity. Nature recycles in ingenious ways. Earlier in this chapter I described the master recycling plan of nature. It made oxidation spontaneous so nothing lives forever, and every bit of the old life is recycled into some parts of the new life. Nature also creates diversity in just as many ways.

THE MASTER SCULPTOR

Anthony's mom may not know this, but the master sculptor is as much at work in the deepest recesses of her muscle cells as it is in the highest reaches of the sky. It shapes and reshapes her muscle cells just as it shapes and reshapes the kaleidoscope of clouds in the sky. Her Type II cells come in three shades: Type IIA, Type IIB and Type IIC. The Type IIC cell is nature's clay. It can align its enzyme machinery to burn fat, or it can realign it to burn sugar. Type IIC muscle cells can change into Type IIA cells and simply burn sugar or they can turn into a Type I cell fitted with fat-burning enzymes. Type IIC cell has its own wisdom. *He* can sense what is required of him. He adapts and adopts, and transforms himself, both in structure and function. He *knows*. The fat-burning enzymes within him also *know*.

UP-REGULATION OF ENERGY DYNAMICS

In scientific terminology, energy is capacity for work. Life is sustained when the chemical bond energy of fats, carbohydrates and proteins is converted into thermal, electromagnetic and mechanical energy for various life functions. During physical exercise, to be more specific, adenosine triphosphate (ATP) is transformed into mechanical injury for muscular contraction. During this process, ATP is degraded either into adenosine diphosphate (ADP) + P + energy or into adenylic acid (AMP) + P + energy. For continued physical activity, ATP must be resynthesized rapidly. This occurs with three distinct molecular pathways: 1) Phosphagen system; 2) Aerobic metabolism when adequate supply of oxygen is readily available; and 3) Anaerobic metabolism when oxygen is not freely available. These basic molecular pathways are schematically shown on the following pages.

I. ENERGY GENERATED WITH PHOSPHAGEN SYSTEM

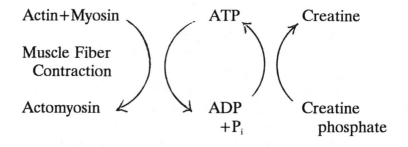

II. ENERGY GENERATED WITH AEROBIC METABOLISM

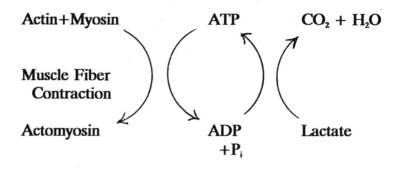

III. ENERGY GENERATED WITH ANAEROBIC METABOLISM

METABOLISM

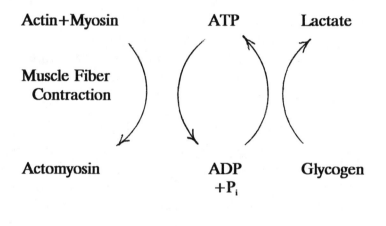

PHOSPHAGEN SYSTEM

The phosphagen system is a system of energy molecules that trigger enzyme fireworks for quick bursts of energy. Phosphagen are molecular packets of ready energy. Nature designed these molecules to support explosive activities — those that require a near-convulsive activity for very short periods of 30 seconds or less. These are the molecules of the initial phases of the so-called fight or flight response. A person or an animal digs his heels to fight for life or takes to his heels for a run for his life.

The primary phosphagen are ATP (adenosine triphosphate) and CP (creatine phosphate). Rich in ready energy, ATP and CP are stored in muscle. They act as match sticks of energy, lighting up the enzyme energy trails as the muscle springs into sudden action. The quarterback enzyme in this reaction is CPK (creatine phosphokinase). It catalyzes resynthesis of ATP as fast as it is utilized. CP stores, however, are limited. Quick starts of sprinters and sudden motions of weight lifters would not be possible without phosphagen molecules. Physical activities that use up the phosphagen packets of ready energy quickly deplete the muscle stores of these molecules and lead to accumulation of lactic acid, one of the principal fatigue molecules. This is nature's way of assuring that our cortical monkeys don't lead us to self-destruct. I think of such nature's prescriptions every time I see an American gladiator limp and groan with sore muscles. Self-flagellation takes many forms. The cortical monkey is an ingenious animal.

The sugar-burning pathways move into action after the initial phase of about 30 seconds and sustain high output energy states for the next few minutes. In the sugar-burning mode, breakdown of one molecule of glycogen in the muscle initially requires one molecule of ATP and results in the production of three molecules of ATP. The three ATP molecules, in turn, generate nine additional ATP molecules and so on. Little explosions of energy for life.

SOURCES OF ENERGY
IN LIMBIC AND CORTICAL EXERCISE

To differentiate between fat-burning and sugar-burning exercises, I include on the next page in table form the percentage points of the source of energy produced in selected types of exercise. The values for energy generated with fat-burning (F/B) exercises are compared with those produced with sugar-burning (S/B) exercises. The zeros represent close approximations. The values in the phosphagen column represent energy available in the form of the principal energy molecule, ATP, and the principal energy enzyme, CPK.

FAT-BURNING AND SUGAR-BURNING ACTIVITIES

Exercise Type	F/B	S/B	Phosphagen
Limbic exercise	95	5	0
Marathon running	95	5	0
Hiking	95	5	0
Cycling (road)	90	5	5
Running (1,500 M)	40	40	20
Swimming	40	40	20
Tennis	10	20	70
Baseball	0	20	80
Sprinting	0	5	95
Weight Lifting	0	5	95

The numbers in the preceding table delineate clearly the difference between the cortical and limbic exercises. They speak eloquently of the physiologic advantages of the limbic mode of energy dynamics over the cortical mode. Activities like weight lifting and sprinting quickly deplete the muscle phosphagen reserves and burn sugar for quick bursts of energy. Evidently, they do nothing to improve the form and function of fat-burning enzymes. Limbic exercise, marathon running and hiking, by contrast, do not touch phosphagen stores, nor do they prompt into action the sugar-burning enzymes to any significant degree.

I have noticed that when I hike with a goal of reaching a point on my trail, I usually return with sore legs. That never happens if I hike without any goal.

This is an illuminating comment from one of my patients in his late sixties. What deeper insight into the inner workings of our enzymes can anyone give us? What greater understanding of the meddlesome capacity of the cortical monkey can there be? The cortical monkey does his *thing* even as we walk far into the woods on a familiar trail. This is the nature of the beast. He sets the goal. The limbic dog suffers even when we walk in silence on a mountain trail.

ALL EXERCISES ARE GOOD EXERCISE

All exercises have beneficial health effects. Golf is good

for the golfer even though golf may not help people lose excess weight. The same holds for tennis. There is the thrill of motion. There is a joy of energy.

A physician colleague complained how food sticks to his body. I asked him why he played tennis. "To win, of course," he responded tersely. Then he frowned at me with quizzical eyes. I changed the subject. There are a lot of good reasons for playing tennis, of course. Losing weight, in my view, cannot be one of them. I used to play tennis. I remember it felt good to wear the whites and walk to the court with a racquet swinging from one arm. It was fun to hit the ball and celebrate the moment. Hitting the ball usually took a second or two. Celebrating the stroke lasted much longer. (My tennis deteriorated as I lost the inclination to run after a ball flying away from me. Without a conscious awareness, I began to wait for the ball to reach me rather than run after it. Also, without conscious awareness, I began to find it harder and harder to find people to play tennis with. The problem was finally resolved when no one would agree to play with me.)

All exercises are good. However, all exercises are not suitable for people who are trying to attain and maintain an optimal weight for their full life spans. Exercise can be *limbic, fat burning* and invigorating. *Or exercise can be cortical, sugar burning* and so often disappointing.

Why doesn't the African tribal runner get tired after a 50 mile ritual run? Why does the American businessman get tired after running one third of a mile on city streets?

Why are Japanese Sumo wrestlers so grotesquely obese even though they exercise regularly and strenuously in order to build their muscles and to maintain a high state of conditioning? Why are long-distance runners thin? Why are weight lifting, tennis or golf not suitable for attaining and maintaining the life span weight? Why are limbic exercises (brisk walking, running or cycling) so suitable for this purpose? The true nature of limbic exercise unfolds before the mind's eye as we reflect upon some common everyday observations about physical activity and fitness. Cortical exercises when performed for weight loss are punitive; limbic exercises are rewarding. Cortical exercises are competitive, hard, highly charged, task-oriented and frequently cause aching. Limbic exercises are indulgent, pampering and easy on our muscles and ligaments.

When an African tribal runner runs on the African savannah, he is running to the beat of some distant drummer. He is linked to a larger something. He has no goals, no stress, no one to impress. He runs, free in body, free in mind and free in spirit.

When an American businessman runs, he is out to get his endorphin high. He has "clever" designs for revitalizing his heart, improving his circulation, raising his pulse to a pre-determined goal set by his cardiologist, lowering his LDL cholesterol, raising his HDL cholesterol, losing his paunch, tightening up his muscles and un-cluttering his mind. And he has all but 17 minutes to *achieve* this. Seventeen minutes! That is all the time he has for meeting his tough goals. How does he do it? By getting fatigued and stressed and frustrated. His muscles ache. His body cries. His thoughts are of anger. His mind is weary. He ends his run tired, tired and aching in body, tired and confused in mind, tired and depleted in spirits, tired and cheated of his endorphin high.

There are several energy and molecular events that occur during slow, sustained exercise. Below I list them, and describe these events. Benefits of general exercises are too obvious to be belabored here. The types of enzymatic up-regulation achievable with limbic exercise listed above are of special importance to us in our pursuit of attaining and maintaining life span weight.

The Molecular Up-regulation
The Myocyte Mitochondrial Up-regulation
The Adipocyte Up-regulation
The Cardiovascular Up-regulation
The Musculoskeletal Up-regulation
The Limbic Up-regulation

THE MOLECULAR UP-REGULATION

I begin this discussion of the fat-burning enzymes with molecular upregulations within the myocyte and the adipocyte to underscore the importance of the many molecular pathways that are normalized by exercise, but that do not relate directly to the function of myocyte or adipocyte.

Perhaps most important of these are the events that lead to functional optimization of various enzyme systems in these cells. I discuss the enhancement of the myocyte and adipocyte enzyme functions in the chapter *On the Nature of Obesity.*

Indeed, the healthful enzymatic effects of exercise have been observed in all enzyme systems studied so far. For instance, superoxide dismutase is one of the first enzymes that protects our tissues from injury caused by free radicals. Physical training increases the activity of this enzyme in the red blood cells (Am J Clin Nutr 51:1093;1990).

Exercise has profound effects on the regulation of one of the primary energy resource molecules of the human frame: the sugar molecule. Non insulin-dependent diabetes is regarded by many physicians specializing in preventive medicine as essentially a disease of sugar overload and physical inactivity. In the chapter On the Nature of Obesity in *The Butterfly and Life Span Nutrition,* I discuss at length the numerous interrelationships between sugar overload, insulin dysfunction, hypertension, Syndrome X of the heart, many cardiovascular and other degenerative disorders.

The problem of molecular damage caused by environmental pollutants is generally ignored in clinical practice. The principal reason for this is the ready access for clinical ecologists to specialized laboratories with capability for necessary testing for pollutants. The absence of firm laboratory data proving the role of pollutants in the cause of clinical disorders has led to the widespread belief among the physician community that this problem does not exist. The ostrich in us loves to bury its head in sand.

While the situation in clinical medicine is generally dismal, the enormous magnitude of this problem is being defined by careful studies in research setting. Consider the following quote.

The results show that their (Polish population) exposure to environmental pollution is associated with significant increase in carcinogen -DNA adducts (PAH-DNA and aromatic adducts), in sister chromatid exchange including high-frequency cells, and in the chromosomal aberrations as well as a doubling in the frequency of ras oncogene overexpression. We found that aromatic adducts on DNA were significantly correlated with chromosomal mutations, providing us with a molecular link between environmental exposure and a genetic alteration relevant to cancer and reproductive risk.

Science 360:256; 1992.

Translation: environmental pollutants are mutilating our genes. They are destroying our enzymes, banishing life.

In the above study, the focus of investigators was on the damage to genes caused by molecules in the family polycyclic aromatic hydrocarbons. My colleagues and I in environmental medicine are equally concerned about the damage done to metabolic and detoxification enzymes by environmental pollutants. Physicians who specialize in environmental medicine about the beneficial effects of slow, sustained exercise for persons with chemical sensitivity and environmental illness. They know that cortical exercises that lead to hyperventilation and sweating are nowhere near as effective in the clinical management of these patients as are the slow, sustained exercise. Of course, limbic exercises bring forth a spiritual dimension that, in my judgement, is essential for good long-term results.

Most environmental pollutants are lipophilic (fat loving) and have long half-lives, several months to several years. It is very difficult to eliminate these toxicants without turning over the fat which binds them tightly. Some of the benefits of exercise in chemical sensitivity appear to accrue from elimination of sweat oils which are rich in environmental toxicants. Other benefits are related to the improved handling of fats in foods by the various metabolic pathways.

It is important to recognize in this context that popular types of exercise that lead to sweating are not as effective in lowering body toxin overload as slow, sustained exercises. The reason for this is obvious. Sweat does not carry fat-loving toxins; increased excretion of skin oils do. *Hence, the optimal exercises for chemical sensitivity and toxicity are slow, sustained exercises that facilitate excretion of sweat oils.*

THE MYOCYTE-MITOCHONDRIAL UP-REGULATION

There are many myocyte-mitochondrial benefits. In the chapter On the Nature of Obesity in the companion volume,

The Butterfly and Life Span Nutrition, I identify two primary biochemical lesions which cause catabolic maladaptation and obesity: mitochondrial enzymatic insufficiency and lipocyte lipase dysfunction. In limbic exercise, our mitochondrial goals are to increase the number of mitochondria, strengthen them and enhance their efficiency. Mitochondria invigorated with limbic exercise function briskly, efficiently and optimally not only during the period of limbic exercise but *at all times.* The benefits of limbic exercise are in bringing these fundamental changes in mitochondrial function. *The primary benefit of limbic exercise is not simply "burning calories."*

UP-REGULATION OF THE FAT CELL

The fat cell is a tiny cell packed with triglyceride fat. Slow, sustained exercise is essential for the health of the adipocyte.

An average adult is estimated to contain about 30 billion adipocytes. These cells are increased both in their number and size in the obese state. Nature designed the adipocyte as a tiny packet of stored energy. Energy is stored in an adipocyte as a tiny droplet of fats. Triglycerides, the main type fat in the fat cells occurs as tiny droplets, about 0.5 microgram in weight. (For comparison, a teaspoon can hold roughly 4 million micrograms of sugar.) An average adult carries about 15 kg (33 pounds) of fat in his 30 billion adipocytes. Since one gram of fat contains 9 calories, it follows that an average adult has 135,000 calories stored in his adipocytes. This depot of energy can sustain an adult through a 40-50 day fast.

A triglyceride molecule is formed by three fatty acids linked together with a single molecule of an alcohol called glycerol. The types of fatty acids included in triglycerides in adipocytes reflect the composition of fatty acids in the diet. Life span foods fill the adipocytes with unspoiled, unoxidized fatty acids; aging-oxidant foods lead to the storage of oxidized fatty acids. Studies have shown that diets rich in life span oils such as oleic acid (olive oil is an important source of this oil) lead to a higher quantity of healthful fatty acids in adipocytes.

The fat cell is an intelligent cell. The wisdom of this cell shows itself in how it orchestrates the workings of the molecules that reside on its surface and those that live within it. There are molecules on its surface that it uses as hooks. It literally fishes for molecules it needs from the soup of life fluids that bathes its surface. These molecules include various hormones and other important "intelligence" molecules of the body. It has its own enzymes, and it has messenger RNA molecules that it uses to make daughter enzyme molecules.

The cell membrane of the fat cell is a marvel of biology.
It separates internal order of a cell from external disorder. It serves as the principal clearing house for the cellular intelligence data. It transforms intelligence data into physical energy and molecular changes. It keeps under surveillance the intrinsic cellular self-destruct mechanisms. It alters its own image and structure to respond to changes in its environments. It serves the cell as its skin, its bowel, its kidneys, its lungs, all rolled in one. It influences the regulatory mechanisms for cellular growth, differentiation and reproductive potential. In

essence, it *thinks* for the cell.

The adipocyte watches out for dangers. It fends for itself. It has sentinel molecules. It has gatekeeper molecules. It has builder molecules and scavenger molecules. It has molecules which it is willing to sacrifice and others which it guards with its life. It has slave molecules and master molecules. It has spies and messengers. The adipocyte has clear ideas of its internal organization, and it is capable of responding and adapting to preserve that order.

LIPASE: THE GUARDIAN MOLECULE

In the fat cell, the lipase enzymes gauge the fat reserves and sense the need for bringing in more fatty acids or putting out more fats. In the capillaries (tiny blood vessels), lipase keeps a sharp eye out for the fat globules that float by. Unlike many of us who indulge in Sunday brunches in choice restaurants, lipase takes only what it knows the cell needs. It breaks up (hydrolyzes) triglycerides in the circulating blood into free fatty acids and glycerol molecules. Fatty acids are pulled into the fat cell for synthesis of the triglycerides as described above.

Human fat cells can make free fatty acids from certain sugars called hexoses, so named because they contain six carbon atoms. These cells can make fatty acids from proteins, though molecular pathways for this are indirect and complex. But the fat cell does not prefer these molecular maneuvers. There is no molecular economy in this. The fat cell likes to keep things simple. It prefers its free fatty acids fresh, uninjured and nontoxic. It sends out the lipase molecules to harvest fresh free fatty acids much like our ancestors used to send their children to their vegetable patches at cooking time.

> *.... weight loss in very obese subjects leads to the increased activity and expression of lipoprotein lipase, thereby potentially enhancing lipid storage and making further weight loss more difficult.*

N Eng J Med 322:1051; 1990

Translation: Dieting is doomed to failure. Our fat-burning enzymes don't have much respect for our dieting gurus. When we simplistically eat less food with dieting to lose weight, the molecular wisdom of lipases in the fat cell senses an impending famine. It *knows* that deliberate attempts are being made to starve the cell it lives in. It *knows* its responsibility. It recognizes it must prepare for a famine. It sees the utter necessity for building up the reserves of the fat cells. It begins its work to hoard fat.

The fat cell also has its own designs for cellular intelligence. It employs porters (lipase enzyme molecules) to carry in more fats for what it suspects might be a time for famine. The fat cell also has a plan B. Afraid that its porters may be waylaid, it generates a whole new team of fatty acid porters by firing up its lipoprotein lipase RNA messenger. Still uncertain, the fat cell has a plan C. It engages in intense motivational seminars for its young porters. The fat cells know how to guard themselves against the folly of dieting.

Exercise up-regulates adipocyte (fat cell) function in many different ways. It increases the sensitivity of the adipocyte cell membrane to insulin. It improves glucose utilization and prevents molecular roller coaster effects. Exercise increases the amount of lipase enzymes and enhances their efficiency. Indeed, all the metabolic roles of adipocytes that I describe in *The Butterfly and Life Span Nutrition* have been examined in the context of physiologic effects of exercise, and show improvement with physical exercise.

THE MUSCULOSKELETAL UP-REGULATION

There are several important benefits that follow the structural and functional up-regulation of the musculoskeletal system. Exercise energizes muscles. It increases the muscle mass. It increases their strength. By putting healthy stress on the bones, it continuously shapes and models bone tissues (the best prevention of osteoporosis). Exercise gives us fluidity and spontaneity in muscle and bone motions. I discuss some aspects of what I call limbic lengthening of muscles, tendons and ligaments in the next chapter.

There is the old saying, "Firm in body, firm in mind." Most of us will dismiss this as childlike trivia. Maybe it is. What is not childlike trivia is that musculoskeletal restrictions develop during the sleep hours in all of us beyond our teen years. The human frame is delicately balanced around the axial skeleton of the neck and torso. There is a pandemic of chronic and back pain in the world today (popularly designated as "subluxation of the vertebrae"). It is, in essence, unbalanced muscular contractions on the two sides of the axial vertebral column. It often starts as an innocuous "tightness in the neck" or "stiffness in the back" which we first notice after sleeping in certain positions. Neglected for long periods of time, it changes into the so-called arthritis in the neck and back. Arthritis in young people, I might add here, is due to autoimmune injury caused by sensitivity to foods, molds, viruses, spirochetes (i.e. Lyme Disease) and bacteria. That may appear to be very simplistic but is based on my extensive personal experience.

MYSTERY OF OBESITY

If there is any mystery about the cause of obesity, it is locked up in the workings of muscle and fat cells.

The muscle cell is the cell where the action begins and the fat cell is where it ends. The study of these two types of cells reveals the true nature of obesity. It is through an understanding of the structure and function of the two cells that we can begin to discern the marvels of biology that keep us lean and energetic. It is also through an understanding of these two cells that we clearly see the utter irrationality of the prevailing ideas of dieting for weight loss. Life span foods nourish these cells; aging-oxidant foods paralyze their life-sustaining enzyme systems. Fat-burning exercises energize their fat-burning enzymes; sugar-burning exercises energize their sugar-burning enzymes. Antibiotics, pesticides and fungicides destroy their enzymes as do toxic metals and industrial pollutants.

Obesity is a problem of emaciated myocytes and bloated adipocytes. Obesity is not a problem of the mind. Dieting is not a solution to the problem of obesity. Those who choose to diet do not know the biology of these cells (or do not choose to learn about these cells for reasons only they understand).

MUSCLE FIBER TYPE AND OBESITY

It seems to me that the entire thrust of our exercise experts is to conduct short term experiments to define, within very narrow limits, a biochemical or structural abnormality which occurs *after* the changes in the weight or muscles have occurred due to poor nutrition and physical inactivity. Such studies are useful in that they enlighten us about molecular or cellular damages associated with these factors. The problem starts when the results of such studies are used to advance the goals of our N^2D^2 medicine.

"The evidence supports the hypothesis that muscle fiber type is an etiological factor for obesity."

Lancet 335:805; 1990

Here is another excellent study which strengthens our grasp of the problem of obesity. Physical inactivity, poor nutrition, toxic foods and dieting cause muscle fiber wasting. Obesity leads to loss of fat-burning muscle fibers.

The above study adds to our knowledge one important sense: It shows a clear inverse relationship between the percentage of body fat and the percentage of fat-burning Type I muscle fibers. As the percentage of body fat increased from about 5% to about 26%, the number of Type I muscle fibers decreased from about 70% to about 10% .

When I read this report, I wondered how long will it take for someone to think of a drug which would increase the number of fat-burning Type I muscle fibers? That would cure obesity for all times, wouldn't it? Another miracle pill. Another triumph for the synthetic chemistry. Another deception. Another skylight.

The authors of the preceding report write,

Metabolic evidence in 50 men, provided by the respiratory exchange ratio (RER) during cycle ergometry, indicated that fatter men (or, in the subset of 11 men, those with a lower proportion of slow muscle fibers) combusted less fat during work at 100 W than did lean men (or those with a high proportion of slow fibers).

Translation: Fat people have sluggish mitochondria and they are inefficient in turning fats into energy. Now is there something in this that we didn't really know about? Is it something that the classical Greeks or Egyptians before them didn't know?

More important, how are we going to use this insight? Are we going to use this insight to help overweight people learn to do limbic exercises? Or are we going to develop a whole new "ergometric" system for exercise to "burn off fat"? A whole new numbering game of fiber type count? Or will we do muscle biopsies on fat men and women to prove that they have lost fat-burning Type I muscle fibers? What next? Blame the muscle fibers? Continue to eat toxic fats? Devise yet another miracle diet? It never fails. Long live numbers.

RAISING THE MUSCLE ANABOLIC SET POINT

There are many physiological benefits of raising the muscle anabolic set point. The most obvious beneficial effect, of

course, is the arrest of excessive muscle catabolism
(breakdown). Dieting decreases muscle mass, the tissues where
fats are burned down (fats are burned down in the muscle). It
decreases the activities of enzymes involved in fat breakdown
and decreases the ability of insulin to break down sugars. It
impairs the sodium and potassium pumps which are essential
for energy generation and decreases the breakdown of stress
and panic molecules produced by biologic stressors.

Increasing the muscle mass, by lowering the muscle
catabolic set point, increases the energy level by reversing all
of the above biologic changes.

THE CARDIOVASCULAR UP-REGULATION

The cardiovascular up-regulation brought about by slow,
sustained exercise far outnumber the benefits of the
conventional ideas of cardiovascular fitness that are based on
the goal of 70% of maximal activity. I personally know of
several deaths caused by misdirected and dangerous infatuation
with driving the muscles and other body organs hard to achieve
some silly numerical goals.

We all recognize the enormous burdens imposed upon
our cardiovascular system by stress, poor nutrition,
environmental pollutants, viruses and autoimmune injury. The
beneficial effects of exercise in the prevention and treatment of
cardiovascular diseases are too well known to be described in

detail here. There is one critically important, but poorly known, aspect of the relationship between exercise and heart disease.

These results support the concept that large changes in weight during young adulthood increase the risk of coronary disease and of cancer.

Am J Epidemiol 129:312; 1989

First, weight fluctuation was most strongly associated with adverse health outcomes in the youngest cohorts (age 30 through 44 years).

N Eng J Med 324:1839; 1991.

I include the preceding citations here for two very important practical reasons. First, a huge number of Americans are exposed to these dangers. Approximately 50 percent of American women and 25 percent of American men diet at any given time (Public Health Service, 1985:2.5. DHHS publication no. (PHS) 86-1250). Second, it is important to emphasize the dangers of dieting programs designed to quickly lose weight and to rapidly "burn off" the calories with exercise without first understanding the real issues and without first going through proper physical training.

THE LIMBIC UP-REGULATION

Finally, there are limbic benefits of limbic exercise. These are the benefits of canceling out the cortical clutter, listening limbically to the body tissues, allowing ourselves some deeply personal time, being kind to ourselves and escaping into limbic openness and new spiritual dimensions. My personal perspective is that these benefits, in the long run, far outweigh the other types of benefits described previously.

I have not been a spiritual man all my life. I can't just become spiritual now that I need it.

Recently, a fifty-year-old executive consulted me for advanced coronary artery disease. He had just returned from a well-known center for cardiac surgery — where, in his words, only the *big* cases are accepted — after a successful quadruple bypass surgery. He followed that with two weeks at a celebrated diet edifice on the West Coast where they teach people to eat a diet that, again in his words, cannot be outdone in terms of cutting more fat out. I discuss the frivolousness of this policy of no fats in food fully in my monograph *Choua, Cholesterol Cats and Chelation*. After listening to him and reviewing his files, I began to outline what I generally recommend for people who consult me for such problems. As I mentioned autoregulation, he raised his hand abruptly. I stopped in mid-sentence to listen to what he urgently seemed to want to say.

"I must tell you, I am one of those who insists on absolute proofs," he blurted.

"That's fine with me," I replied calmly.

"I have never been a spiritual person," he added tersely.

"But I am! I mean, I am drawn to things spiritual," I tried to lighten the conversation.

"I really mean it. I am not a spiritual person," he insisted.

"I understand," I tried to back off.

We were silent for a while. I felt his wife's intense eyes fixed on me.

"There are some methods of self-regulation, some ways of breathing that are very helpful," I changed the subject.

"Doc, I must be candid with you. With me, you have to prove everything."

"Proving everything may not be destined for us humans," I tried to make light of our conversation.

"Doc, you don't understand. I have not been a spiritual man. I have spent my life like that. I can't just become spiritual just because I need it," he said, softening up a bit.

Why not? I wondered. People who suffer from advanced heart disease need to understand some things. Their lives depend upon them. Heart disease is not a plumbing problem, though our cardiac surgeons insist it is.

MOON GODDESS SELENE'S HORSE AND GHORAA

The sight of a runner on a sidewalk often takes my thought to Elgin's Marbles. The runner usually looks bored. He is panting for breath. His face is frequently distorted with exertion and anguish. Then I see the face of one of the horses of Moon Goddess Selene.

The first time I saw the statue of Moon Goddess Selene among Elgin's marbles in London, I was stunned by the sheer energy of this horse, struggling to break through the marble in which it was incarcerated over 25 centuries ago. Of course, the horse manifests the craft of some long forgotten master stone-carver. But here in the stillness of a cavernous exhibit hall of the British Museum, I was not overcome by the sculptor's craft. Rather, it was the raw, uncontrollable energy of the beast pitched against the unending punishment of the run. The inscription below the marble piece read,

"The horse is weary from its night-long labor, the eyes bulge, nostrils flare and the mouth gapes as the beast gasps for breath."

Then I remembered I saw the Ghoraa running, limbically,

rhythmically, gracefully and with total abandon. The two horses belong to two different worlds.

Selene is the goddess of sleep. Her horses are mythical horses. But the Greeks knew their gods. They also knew the horses of their gods. They saw in their gods what they saw in the life around them. The Greeks knew some things about the human condition. They understood captivity, conflict and struggle for relief. The anguish of the horse was the anguish of the god struggling for escape.

Elgin's Marbles are really not Elgin's. In the Louvre, the French call them Marbre Pentelique. The Greeks built the Parthenon on the Acropolis to honor their wisdom and peace Goddess Athena, daughter of Zeus, the protector of palace and citadel. They built a massive statue for her and surrounded her with their marbles. A thousand years later, Christians turned the temple into a church. Another thousand years later, the Turks conquered Athens and converted the church into a mosque. In 1687 the Venetian General, Francesco Morosini, laid siege to the Acropolis. The Turks were using the Parthenon as a power magazine. The Parthenon sustained a direct hit from a Venetian shell. The resulting explosion left the Parthenon in shambles. During the early nineteenth century, Thomas Bruce, seventh Earl of Elgin brought these marbles to England. Some Briton, in some delusional plausibility, dubbed the marbles Elgin's Marbles.

Selene's horse reminded me of the anguished faces of a thousand American sidewalk runners with contorted faces, stooping shoulders, cramping legs and heavy feet. The running of the runner has something of Selene's horse in him, captivity within his skin, conflict with fat under his skin, a struggle to drop those messy pounds. There is no relief. The fat takes forever to melt a little. The pounds return in days. The struggle continues. The limbic dog bites, not because he wants to but because he doesn't know any better.

THE HEART OF A RUNNER
VERSUS
THE HEART OF A BODYBUILDER

Who has a bigger heart, a runner or a weight lifter? Who has a healthier heart, a runner or a weight lifter? Who has less risk of developing high blood pressure? A runner or a weight lifter? The correct answer to all three questions is the runner. Why? Almost all types of exercise have beneficial cardiovascular effects. Exercise improves heart function and increases heart size. Compared with matched controls, competitive athletes have a 15% to 20% increase in the thickness and about a 45% increase in the mass of the left ventricle, the heart chamber that pumps the blood to the body (JACC 7:190; 1986). The capacity of the left ventricle to hold blood before it pumps it to the body (end-diastolic dimension) increases by about 10%.

However, not all exercise has equally beneficial

cardiovascular effects. The changes in the heart musculature caused by exercise also depend upon whether the exercise is isotonic (muscular contraction is accompanied by motion) or isometric (muscular contraction is not accompanied by motion). The hearts of weight lifters, who do isometric exercises that primarily put pressure stress on the heart, become stronger and larger in proportion to the strength and size of other muscles. The hearts of runners, who do isotonic exercises that put volume stress on the heart, by contrast, become much larger (and functionally stronger) than those of weight lifters. The reason for this phenomenon is simple: The heart of the bodybuilder *knows* that all it has to do is sustain intense muscular activity for a few moments at a time, while the heart of a runner *knows* it has to support the body tissues for long periods of time. The two hearts change in their size and power in response to the demands imposed upon them.

It may be added here that weight lifters who primarily limit themselves to weight lifting exercise — isometric exercises that are almost exclusively sugar-burning in nature — run a higher risk of hypertension and its complications than persons who do not exercise at all.

HORMONAL UP-REGULATION

Slow, sustained exercise fundamentally changes the state of metabolism and energy. The African tribal messengers knew this. The Greeks and Romans knew this. The Aztecs knew this.

And we know this. The ancients understood well, intuitively it seems, the essential relatedness among tissues. Purely from a rational standpoint, one could argue that exercise must change the hormonal dynamics in the body in a global sense. This indeed is true.

Today, our science and technology allow us to recognize the molecular relatedness in human biology in measurable and reproducible ways. Measurement and reproducibility, of course, is the language of science. Exercise initially causes the release of some stress hormones such as adrenaline (and its cousin molecules, catecholamines) and cortisol. It also leads to release of other hormones such as growth hormone and prolactin. It is well known among the general public that blood levels of certain opiods (beta endorphin, beta lipotropin and others) rise during physical exercise. These hormones have many recognized benefits in areas of sleep, thermoregulation (temperature control in tissues), sexual functions and pain modulation. These are marvels of molecular wisdom. Stress hormones are released to up-regulate the metabolic and energy state of the body; opiods are simultaneously put out to provide a molecular counterbalance — the dis-ease causing aspects of stress hormones are held in abeyance.

THE PLEASURE PILLS

Now a word about runner's high. Our exercise experts thrive on preaching about the bounties of beta-endorphins.

Everyone now knows that these hormones are joy-bars — tiny pleasure pills. What is not generally recognized that these effects wear off with endurance training, and actual amounts of these substances in blood and tissues diminish after exercise in people who run long distances for several years. What does this mean? If we run to win pills of pleasure, there will be no more pills to be found after a while. If not through beta-endorphin, one might ask, how does the African tribal message runner continue to get his high? I suspect it has something to do with the way the sculptor in the sky shapes and reshapes his clouds up above or the hills on the horizon.

There are other marvels of biology in this picture. The heart chambers called atria have supremely crafted sensors that assess the fullness of the blood stream. They serve as sentinels and send warning signals to protect us from the heady demands of our cortical monkey during exercise. Some cells in the atria produce a hormone called atrial natriuretic factor (ANF) when the walls of these chambers are stretched by the rush of blood through them during exercise. This hormone regulates the function of kidneys, facilitates removal of excess salt from the body, normalizes blood pressure, and regulates the state of hydration. A fascinating facet of this hormone is its influence on pituitary which has receptors for it. Some future researchers, I am confident, will unravel this mystery.

THE HEART: A PUMP OR A GLAND?

When I first learned about the ANF, my thoughts drifted

to a debate that took place about 2,500 years ago between two Greek philosophers. Hippocrates, the father of medicine, believed that the human tissues had an innate healing capacity which he called the *physis* — the origin of the word physician. If the injured tissues are allowed to heal, he taught his pupils, they will heal by their inner healing power. An opposing viewpoint was vehemently advanced by Democratis, a contemporary of Hippocrates. Democratis considered Hippocrates's physis a figment of imagination. Human beings, he ridiculed Hippocrates, were nothing but masses of tiny particles which he called atoms. In his philosophy of *atomism,* there was no room for spontaneous recovery brought forth by the injured tissues themselves.   For centuries, the followers of Hippocrates promoted their notion of *vitalism* while the disciples of Democratis fiercely opposed them in support of their idea of *atomism*. This debate has continued ever since.

The ideas of atomism gained greater currency among physicians with passing centuries —   and, with time, they assumed great healing powers over injured tissues. They called their profession the *healing* profession, and bestowed upon themselves the title of *healers.* In eighteenth-century America, Dr. Benjamin Rush,   a physician-signer of the American Declaration of Independence, took sides with Democratis, and expressed the dominant medical philosophy of his day. He wrote,

> *"....., yet in practice they (physicians) are the masters of nature ... , art should take the business (of healing) out of her hands (nature)."*

Italics added

Such assumptions of power on the part of physicians amuse me. And then I think about how physicians of the future might look with amusement at our current ideas of health and disease. It is a humbling thought.

What is a heart? I was taught in medical school that the heart is a pump, a mere pump made up of flesh. The poet, the medical party line continued, may take liberties with what the heart is and what it can do, but the scientist in medicine must be above all such frivolity. Now it turns out that the heart *is* a glandular organ. It does *sense* what flows through it. It does *respond* to events that take place within it. It is not simply a pump. I wonder what Democratis would have thought about it.

****

In closing this chapter, I enumerate most of the well-established physiologic benefits of exercise.

A. Changes Due to Anaerobic Exercise

Up-regulation of enzymes of the phosphagen and anaerobic glycolysis energy systems
Increased tolerance of lactic acid
Increased stores of ATP and CP
Increase in the thickness of the heart muscle

B. Changes Due to Aerobic Exercise

Up-regulation of enzymes that oxidize fats and glycogen

Increased oxidative capacity for fats and glycogen
Increased availability of fats and glycogen
Increased size and number of mitochondria
Increased cavity size of the heart chamber

C. General Changes Due to Exercise

Increased cardiovascular system capacity
Increased total blood volume
Decreased blood pressure
Decreased cholesterol and triglycerides
Increased lean body mass
Decreased total body fat
Increased total hemoglobin
Increased heat acclimatization

We can do exercise for all the benefits of exercise I enumerate here. Or we can exercise for up-regulating our fat-burning enzymes. Or we can exercise limbically, free of all burden of goals, free of need to know. We can experience the exhilaration of motion for motion's sake. We can do so to seek communion with that larger *presence* that surrounds us, with the limbic language of silence.

Chapter 5

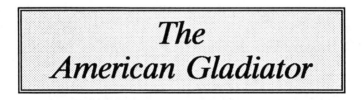

There is an American gladiator out there.

The American gladiator is pledged to fitness. He is totally, completely, utterly pledged to fitness. He is committed to exercise, and his commitment is absolute.

The gladiator knows all the *right* stuff about exercise and fitness. He knows all the right numbers for the tensile strength of his muscles, the percentage points for his exercise physiology and the right Max VO_2 value for his weight and height. He has committed to his mind the chart of split times — so he can quickly determine the precise pace for running to the precise running time he wants. He carries a running diary to keep track of his running data — speed, mileage, weather conditions and the effect of his run on his weight and spirits. He is up-to-date on current guidelines of the American College of Sports Medicine.

The gladiator knows all about the required glycogen stores in his liver and muscles, the needed carbohydrate load in his food, and the right plan for maximizing the benefits of his exercise schedule. He knows all the muscle groups in his body, and can readily name all the individual muscles that bulge when he exercises.

The gladiator knows well the latest inventions of the Star Wars medicine for exercise equipment, the steppers, the striders, the skiers and the swimming machines. He knows all about the most orthopedically *correct* thigh thinners, leg loopers, back blippers, and masseter masters. He excels in rock-climbing in mid-town gyms.

The gladiator is an expert of exercise gear, compression shorts — spandex and all, the resilience of the heels of his running shoes and the toe strength of his walking shoes. He knows the precise chemical composition of the sweat he puts out during exercise. And what fluids he must drink to replenish these losses.

The gladiator's whole philosophy of life is emblazoned on his T-shirt: Doing the hard things the *hardest* way. He is a man of few words. He likes the hardest way because maximal physical stress, he believes, is essential for the maximal achievement. His body parts are often smeared with Ben-gay. A head band distinguishes this martyr as he weaves through the common folks scurrying to their work places.

The American gladiator is defiant. He defies the boredom of exercise. He defies the pain that his exercise brings him. Sometimes he admits his shins cringe with pain as if railroad spikes have been driven into them. (And they are.) Sometimes he speaks of torn ligaments, sometimes of ruptured tendons. His flesh sears with anguish. His heart pounds. His lungs toil to bring in some air of relief. His skin is wet with sweat. But the gladiator goes on. He must, for to stop for him is to die. He is at war.

The gladiator knows all about endorphin highs. He knows when — after 21 minutes — and how — through receptors at the cell membrane — his nerve cells unleash their stores of endorphins, the pleasure molecules. When he is not performing his rituals of fitness, he lives in their memory.

The American gladiator is at war. He knows it. People around it know it. War against what? That's not clear to him nor those around him. He is not alone in this. He has a trainer — a keeper — who goads him along, sometimes cheering him, at others scolding him. The gladiator's keeper is an expert of all matters of exercise. He is well-versed with his exercise charts, the bar graphs of muscle energy, the pie graphs for respiratory functions and the monograms for cardiovascular fitness. He is sharp with his numbers and fast with his tongue. It isn't easy for the keeper either. For if the gladiators give up, his keeper loses his lease on his arena. Without a lease, where would he keep his equipment? Who would want his used iron horses and sweat-smeared electronic skiffs and stained swimming machines. It's a tough world out there. The keeper also lives a tough life.

THE CHOLESTEROL GLADIATORS

In our hospitals, there is another kind of gladiator, the cholesterol gladiator.

This gladiator is a physician. He talks eagerly and intensely about his new exercise program. He is sprung into action by a blood test that shows high cholesterol or triglycerides levels. Sometimes he is shocked into action by a death from heart disease or stroke in the family. He is up on all the statistics of heart disease, all the numbers for hypertension, all the percentage points of risk factors for stroke. He talks about a new determination, a new training gear, a new pair of running shoes. His conversation becomes animated when he talks about his Max VO$_2$ and 70 percentile of his maximum heart rate, correct for his age. He knows an awful lot about the optimal muscular conditioning and cardiovascular fitness. Exercise to him is a precise science, no different from the precise science of drug medicine that he practices. And, of course, he talks about the joys of runner's high. I listen to such conversation with great interest but I don't say anything.

Within some weeks, and rarely after a few months, I see him limping in the hospital parking lot. "A little setback," he speaks with a smile as he responds to his peers when they acknowledge his limp with sympathetic eyes. Some more days pass. His sprained ligaments and tendons do not heal. The knots in his muscles persist. Now he gives hesitant explanations of why his limbs do not move the way they used to. "The years have taken their toll," he concludes.

It is a mundane sight for me now. I have seen surgeons limping in the hospital corridors. I have seen internists limp from their exercise injuries. And, of course, I have seen orthopedists and physiotherapists do it. Muscles, tendons and ligaments don't seem to favor any medical specialty, nor do they carry any bias against another group. The cortical monkey drives them all hard. The bites of the limbic dog are equally sharp for all of them.

THE QUIET INTERNIST

One of the internists in our hospital always keeps silent

when the conversations move to the subject of exercise. It's not that he doesn't like to talk. He is a conservative Republican and is well known for his diatribes against the shenanigans of "those liberal Democrats". He is very thin. On many occasions, I see his plate brimming with food at lunch and hear someone remark how he stays so thin while he eats so much. He usually smiles and mutters something noncommittal about it all being in the genes.

The fat-burning enzymes do not much care for simplistic notions about genes and body fat. I had a sense that there was more to the story of this internist. One day he asked me how my exercise book was coming along. That gave me an excuse to enquire about his exercise routine. He flashed his usual smile and shrugged his shoulders. I pressed him for an answer, and this once he relented. He told me he did do "something." I asked him why he never talked about it.

"What's there to talk," he evaded my question.
"But you do exercise, don't you?" I pressed him.
"Yeah! But it's nothing."
"So tell me what is it?"
"I run," he admitted, as if to a misdemeanor.
"How often?"
"It's nothing." He became evasive again.
"How often do you run?" I persisted.
"Every day."
"How much?"
"I really don't know?"
"You don't know?" I feigned surprise.
"It's really nothing. Maybe a mile! Maybe a mile and a half! I run slowly." He spoke slowly as if to apologize.
"That's great, Ed." I didn't want him to stop.

"Oh, it's nothing. I mean I don't take my pulse. I don't do any breathing counts. I even don't know what my Max VO$_2$ should be. Or what 70% of my maximal rate should be." He stopped.

"Go on, I am listening," I prodded him.

"I don't even run for any specific time or distance. There is really nothing for me to say on exercise. I mean people know so much about exercise. I know nothing about it."

I understood why he remains thin even though he seems to eat freely. His fat-burning enzymes are upregulated. I also understood how he can run every day of the week. Because he runs the way I do, limbically. Limbically like my ghoraa.

THE IRONHORSE GLADIATORS

One day it occurred to me that I should consult some medical texts about exercise. The very thought amused me. How many people would try to write a book about exercise without consulting some medical texts on exercise? I walked over to the hospital library, shaking my head at myself all the way. The library staff had always been so supportive. They pulled out two textbooks on exercise and two other volumes on physical fitness. I opened one of them, *The Orthopedic Clinics of North America*, April 1983, and thumbed through it in a cursory way. My eyes were captured by a photograph on page 444. The caption below the photograph read,

A swimmer can duplicate his strokes on an isokinetic bench.

It was a picture of a balding, obese man strung out on an inclined black metal contraption, his neck strained and lifted off the metal rod beneath his breast bone, his arms extending downwards to reach two stirrups clutched by his hands, his lips pursed, his brow wrinkled. His face grimaced. His silent eyes bore eloquent testimony to the misguided inventiveness of those who built this abominable piece of *fitness* equipment, and the mindless subservience to this equipment of our exercise "experts" who foist them upon innocent, unsuspecting victims of Star Wars medicine.

Why would anyone give up swimming in real water for being strung out on some lifeless metal contraption, I wondered? How could anyone in his right mind substitute the spontaneity of motion in real water with false motions of limbs and torso on a machine? How could anyone trade exhilaration of true-to-life motion for scrutiny of faked movements of his muscles by some exercise expert? The American gladiator and his keeper do not like to answer questions like these. The author of the article continued,

" .... gym consists of a rolling platform that moves up and down on an adjustable inclined plane. .... can do a wide variety of exercises on this apparatus, employing the rolling sled with or without a cable-and-pulley assembly."

I read these lines and my eyes drifted back to the picture of the bald man strung out on the abominable contraption which its inventor chose to call a swimming machine. Why has common sense become so uncommon in medicine, I wondered?

THE SPEEDWALKING GLADIATOR

After I finished one of my exercise workshops for my patients, two men and a woman approached me. The older of the two men appeared to be in his early fifties. He had heard me discuss limbic breathing on one of Dr. Robert Atkins' WOR radio shows in New York. He thought limbic breathing might give him an edge during speed walking races, and came to learn it along with two of his speed walking companions. During the preceding months, he told me, he had been losing his speed. His toes were not pushing the way they used to. His leg muscles cramped during the race. He was deeply distressed about these problems, and, of course, that increased his stress problem. He spoke with great intensity. He was determined, he insisted repeatedly, to regain his lost power and speed.

I wondered how I was going to break the news to him that limbic breathing and limbic exercise are about escaping the cortical clutches. The limbic state is about yielding, listening and, yes, receiving. It is not about competing. I shouldn't have worried. The gladiator in the speed walker was not into listening. He had already figured out how he was going to use limbic breathing to resolve his speed walking problems. He didn't need any affirmation from me. He asked me several questions but didn't seem eager to wait for my answers. He spoke his piece, triumphantly looked at his companions and walked out. The American gladiator is into doing things. He is not into listening.

I CANNOT HELP COMPETING WITH MYSELF

Jennifer, a woman in mid-thirties, consulted me for incapacitating chronic fatigue of two years duration. She gave me a fairly typical clinical history of so-called chronic fatigue syndrome. She had suffered from multiple allergies all her life, from eczema, milk intolerance and urticaria (hives) in infancy, from nasal congestion, sinusitis and recurrent sore throats in her childhood, and from sensitivity to detergents, solvents and formaldehyde during her adult years. Her allergies had remained undiagnosed and her recurrent infections were treated with multiple courses of antibiotics.

During the two years previous to her visit with me, she developed the classical full-blown clinical picture of chronic fatigue with muscle aches and cramps, abdominal bloating and cramps, undue sensitivity to cold, and problems of mood, memory and mentation. Along the way she developed some chest symptoms, and her cardiologist promptly gave her the diagnosis of mitral valve prolapse. (Mitral valve prolapse, I might add here to reassure readers who have been given this diagnostic label, is nothing more than a state of molecular hypervigilance that stresses the heart and creates the artifact of mitral valve prolapse on echocardiogram. What these individuals desperately need is training in how to slow their hearts and cure the prolapse. Instead, they are given beta blocker drugs. Rare examples of rheumatic fever injuring the mitral valve and causing prolapse, of course, are exceptions.)

"I can't get out of my bed in the morning,"

Jennifer told me during her first visit. Jennifer made very satisfactory — and entirely predictable — recovery with diagnosis and treatment of her mold, pollen and food allergy, oral and intravenous nutrient therapies, autoregulation and some limbic exercise. During a follow-up visit about 3 months after her initial consultation, she talked excitedly about her recovery and asked me if I would help her tackle the next problem: She was about 65 pounds overweight. I put her on very low carbohydrate diet that I have had good results with in clinical cases similar to that of Jennifer. She had attended my workshop on limbic exercise which helped me in prescribing an exercise program for her. Specifically, I underscored the need for slow and sustained exercise for up-regulating her fat-burning enzymes. Exercise that will cause you to break in sweat and hyperventilate, I repeated for emphasis, will be sugar-burning exercise, and one cannot up-regulate fat-burning enzymes with sugar-burning exercise. She seemed to understand all this fully and left with evident enthusiasm.

During the next visit about a month later she told me she had lost five pounds. I asked her to describe to me how she did her exercise and what benefits she obtained from them. She talked about how good she felt after she broke into sweat during the exercise. "But Jennifer, that's not what we had discussed," I protested, "that's not all what I prescribed for you specifically." She sensed the disappointment in my voice and said,

> *"Ali, all my life I have been competitive. I can't help but compete with myself. Dr. Ali, for two years I couldn't get out of my bed. I guess now I am trying to make up for the lost time."*

The gladiator is a child of the cortical monkey. It dies hard.

THE CHEMISTRY OF DOING THINGS
THE HARDEST WAY

Lactic acid is one of the important fatigue molecules. In health, production of lactic acid is balanced with its consumption. During normal activity, muscles and other body organs produce lactic acid, and the liver and kidneys consume it. During exercise, production of lactic acid increases sharply. When sufficient oxygen is not available, all tissues produce lactic acid. Normally, lactic acid is converted into another acid called pyruvic acid which, in turn, is oxidized to produce energy and build high-energy ATP energy molecules from low-energy ADP and AMP molecules.

Lactic acid is also a cul-de-sac molecule. During limbic exercise, the utilization of lactic acid for energy purposes proceeds evenly and there is no build-up of either this acid or its breakdown product, pyruvic acid. Cortical exercises disrupt this balance. When sufficient oxygen is not available to break down lactic and pyruvic acids, both accumulate and increase acidotic and oxidative stress on tissues. Flow of electrons (tiniest packets of energy) through the cytochrome enzyme system is slowed down, and the generation of high-energy ATP molecules is impaired. As a result, the low-energy ADP and AMP molecules accumulate. All these changes lead to activation of an enzyme (phosphofructokinase) that plays a central role in the breakdown of sugar stored in the liver and muscle as glycogen. The acidotic and oxidative stresses on the tissues so produced bring to a halt any further activity. Lactic acid, pushed to the corner, shifts the total energy chemistry of energy into a slower gear so that molecular recovery can take place.

Nature has built into our energy metabolism some safety nets. These nets, it seemed to have reasoned, will become necessary to prevent self-inflicted damage. The American gladiator is a defiant animal. He pushes and pushes. He likes to do the hard things the *hardest way.* The tissues accumulate pools of lactic acid. ATP is depleted. ADP and AMP builds up. Energy mechanisms come to a halt. The tissues begin to drown in pools of ADP and AMP, and send distress signals. The gladiator pushes himself harder and harder. His keeper pushes him harder still. The tissues are deprived of oxygen and nourishment. The cells bloat with waste. The muscles cry out in pain. The heart palpitates. The lungs struggle. The gladiator goes on and on in his death-defying dance of fitness.

EXERTIONAL RHABDOMYOLYSIS

The word rhabdo refers to the type of muscle that is under our voluntary control (skeletal or striated muscle fibers). The term myolysis means breakdown. Thus, the term exertional rhabdomyolysis means *death of muscle cells.* Little does the gladiator realize that his death-defying fitness crusade, in reality, brings death to his muscle cells.

The muscle cells bustle with activity during exercise. The Ph decreases and the temperature increases; both factors improve delivery of oxygen to the cell innards by decreasing oxygen affinity of hemoglobin (by displacing oxygen off hemoglobin molecules). The enzymatic actions in the muscle cells lead to generation of mediator molecules that further facilitate the metabolic actions of minerals such as potassium in ionic (electrically charged) form. These molecular events lead to vasodilatation — the blood vessels in the tissues open up to let in the nourishment and facilitate removal of cellular waste.

All of this, of course, is the natural order of things. It keeps energy enzymes in peak performance. What happens when the cortical monkey overdrives the tissues? Lactic acid accumulates. Cell sap becomes acidotic. Oxyradicals overwhelm the free radical quenchers and poke holes in the cell membrane. The cell innards hemorrhage. The cells dies. Melodrama! Not really. Studies of athletes engaged in endurance training clearly show evidence of cell injury and cell death. Blood levels of some enzymes such as LD (lactic dehydrogenase) and CK (creatine kinase) rise in people after muscle trauma from accidents and in patients with muscle disorders called myopathies.

Sudden death has been documented among marathon runners during the run. In a few such cases when autopsy was performed, the pathologists found death of a large number of individual heart muscle cells. The gladiator regularly kills his muscle cells but is told by his trainer that is good. It is only after you injure the muscle cells that they grow stronger, so goes the wisdom among some circles devoted to sculpting muscles.

THE CARDIOVASCULAR GLADIATOR

Diane, a woman in early sixties, is receiving chelation therapy for advanced heart disease. She has undergone bypass surgery twice, each time with poor results. She is satisfied with the clinical improvement she has seen with chelation treatment. Her husband, however, is not comfortable with such therapy. "If chelation therapy was any good, why wouldn't all the cardiologists in the country do it?" he often confronts his wife. She talked to me about it once. Of course, this argument is not new for holistic physicians. If nutritional medicine really works, I have been asked many times, why don't all doctors do it? The answer is really simple: When the physicians are required to practice preventive medicine, they will practice nutritional medicine. At present, they are required to practice drug medicine only, and that is what they do. As for chelation therapy versus cardiac surgery, there is no contest. There is more than $100,000 in every operation for the cardiac center and the surgeon. Chelation therapy will barely bring them $3,000.

During one recent visit, she told me about an episode of chest pain during her exercise at the cardiac rehabilitation center. I recognized the obvious danger in that sort of exercise. Every physician knows of fatal heart attacks triggered by stressful exercise. I asked her if she did exercise in the slow and sustained way I had taught her.

"I started doing it your way, Dr. Ali, but .... " she stopped in mid-sentence.

"But what?" I asked.

"My husband thinks it is silly," she answered apologetically.

"Silly?" I was taken aback.

"My cardiologist also agrees with my husband," she added.

"But what is silly?" I was now very curious.

"They think it is silly. They are pretty sure it can't work if doesn't push the heart rate up," she answered.

"Silly!" I murmured to myself.

"They think it is silly to expect any benefits from what you call limbic exercise. They think you have to exercise hard enough to push your heart rate for cardiovascular fitness."

"Push hard even when that causes chest pain?" I asked incredulously.

"I know it doesn't seem right but that's what my cardiologist has prescribed. And my husband won't have it any other way."

"You have to be careful. Chest pain during exercise is a clear danger signal." I expressed my concern."

"I know! I know! But you know my husband is not all that thrilled about the chelation treatment. I don't want to push my luck. I figure I will do chelation here and do exercise their way."

The cardiovascular gladiator is not to be messed with. He loves his percentage points. Subtract your age from 220, he speaks with an authoritative voice, and then multiply that number by 70 percent to find your maximal heart rate. Sometimes he raises his demands and pushes the percentage all the way up to 90 percent. Next, it is the turn of a gladiator from

Canada. The Canadian gladiator mercilessly reviles the American. The correct number, he pronounces with overriding authority is 209 minus 60 percent of the age. And that's not all. For cyclists, he declares with finality, the true number is 205 minus 60 percent of the age. Long live the gladiator! Long live his percentages!

WHO'S WINNING? IT DOESN'T MATTER

Winning is not everything, Vince Lombardi exclaimed. Winning is the only thing, he pronounced.

Two men were playing chess on a street. A passerby walked by and then turned around to watch the chess game. He studied the board for a while and then asked, "Who is winning?" The chess players didn't respond. The passerby observed the game in silence for some more minutes and then asked again, "Who is winning?" Again, there was no response from the chess players. The man studied the chess board for some more time, and repeated his question for the third time. One of the chest players looked up and tersely replied, "It doesn't matter."

YOU WON! NOW WE WILL WALK BACK

One day, Talat and I turned from Broadway on to 73rd

street on our way to Schwab House. At about the middle of the block, two little boys, barely five years in age, sprinted past us. Several yards from us, one of the boys came to a sudden halt. His face was flushed, with tiny beads of sweat glistening on his pink forehead. His curly blond hair almost completely covered his left eye. He leaned forward and rested his little pink hands on his knees, reducing the obvious tremor in his tissues. The second boy broke his sprint, stopped a few yards ahead of the first one and then slowly walked back to his companion, grinning with a winner's smile. The first boy grinned broadly as the winner neared him, and shook his head in conceding victory to his friend. As we came upon them, I heard the first boy say with evident joy, "You won! Now we will walk back." Who won? Who lost? I wondered.

Lombardi's words, I have been told, speak for the quintessential American experience. They resonate in the deepest recesses of the American psyche. We are a nation of winners, we are told as we grow up. It seems just the right prescription for raising our children, a grand design to sustain our national pride. The right stuff for our national hopes and dreams. I sometimes wonder about Lombardi's words. Is winning really the only thing?

We Americans have been a winning people. Or so the slogan goes. We split the atom. We dropped the bombs and taught the Japanese a thing or two. In the 1950s and 1960s, we were intoxicated with our power. The greatest power that ever existed, we crooned, with good reasons. If we could reach the moon, we exulted, we could reach the stars. When we set our minds to anything, we asked our children to repeat after us, we can do everything.

We thrived on cold war. Russians threatened to bury us, but we knew better. God was on our side. We could afford guns as well as butter. Riots in Watts seemed an anomaly. Newark burned, but that was subversion by the Un-Americans amongst us. Some folks living in the Ironbound section of Newark were safe: Their community leaders had the courage to wave their guns and taunt the rioters. "Com'n! Try us. We will shoot you down like rabbits. We will shoot first and ask questions later." The whole country saluted them — for a fine display of the finest American tradition.

We built a grand illusion. As individuals, we could be deprived, angry and impoverished, and yet, as a people, we were going to win. And winning, our prophet Lombardi told us, was the only thing.

The planet Earth shrank into a global village. Some of us saw that, but the Lombardies in America won. Winning was the only thing.

As individuals, we got angrier and angrier. It didn't matter how deeply troubled we were as individuals, as American people we were winners. After all, winning — our prophet Lombardi had taught us — was the only thing. And clearly America was winning. Japanese were fussing with their electronic trinkets, but we had our Big Blue. Detroit was invincible. Watts and Newark were anomalies. We were winners. And winning was not everything, it was the only thing.

We Americans were a playing people. We were not a nation of mere observers. We Americans made things happen. We did not simply watch things happen. Competition was the name of our game. Winning was the only thing.

Winning is the only game in town. The folks at the FDA are Americans. For them too, winning is not everything, it is the only thing. The FDA knows its charge: to protect uninformed Americans from the charlatans in healthcare. It is determined to meet its responsibility head on. The year it banished the use of tryptophan for those who suffered from depression, the makers of Prozac rang in a billion dollars. How many people were hurt by tryptophan? A dozen? Two dozens? How many thousands continue to be hurt by Prozac? The gladiators at the FDA are not interested in such questions. Now they propose to classify vitamins and minerals as drugs if dosage exceeds what *their* scientists have determined to be the recommended daily allowance. What can we expect if these FDA warriors do succeed? I take 5,000 to 6,000 mg of vitamin C as my daily supplement. Since the RDA value of vitamin C is 60 mg — and the tablet size will be expected to be 60 mg — I will need to write myself a prescription for 3,000 tables for every month. So will I need to do for my patients. How much will those prescriptions cost me? And my patients? Who will profit from this? Winning is not everything for the gladiators at the FDA. It is the only thing.

THE BATTLE OF BREASTS

One community hospital I know spent close to a million

dollars on a marketing blitz. They told women they had a better mousetrap for diagnosing breast cancer. TV sells, they knew. Glossy, colorful brochures are expensive, but they do bring in the *beef*. And so it happened. They increased their "breast market share". The other hospitals in the community could not simply let their breast market share be stolen from them. They rose in defense of their breast market share. They all responded with winning strokes. Their brochures were prettier, their ads more glamorous. A fierce battle of breasts was waged. Before the dust settled on the battle field, a $175.00 diagnostic biopsy for breast cancer changed into a $550.00 service. Who won? Who lost? All the hospitals moved on to some other bigger and better battles — winning games as they call it. The folks in our hospitals are Americans. We Americans are a winning people. And winning is not everything. It is the only thing for us.

Los Angeles burned again. A jury told us that what we saw on a video dozens of time wasn't what we really saw on that video. A man on the ground convulsed with pain as four men hit him with clubs 32 times — or was it 52 times? What we saw on video was discipline in the process of enforcement — a kind of justice. My father, a judge, told me many years ago that justice is blind. I wondered if that is what he meant. The week Los Angeles burned, someone told me a gladiator was awarded a multimillion dollar contract for playing ball. Long live our gladiators! And long live their keepers!

We are a more somber America now. Most of us are hurting now. Many of us are beginning to see the false promise of our false prophet. We Americans cannot grow angrier and angrier as individuals and yet hold on to the grand dream of greatness as a people. We can be only as rich as the poorest among us. We Americans can be only as rich as the poorest

among the people of this global village. We think of the teeming
billions crammed into a polluted, shrinking planet Earth. We
look at our children and wonder: Is there hope?

A BLIND WOMAN IN A SNOWSTORM

A legally blind woman was getting ready to leave the
office during a heavy snowstorm. She could barely see things
some feet ahead of her. The office staff was worried how she
was going to walk unescorted to her apartment some blocks
away from the office in a blinding snowfall. They volunteered to
call a taxi. She declined, wrapped herself in her long coat and
a shawl, and stepped out. I saw her go out and wondered about
human senses and sensibilities.

The blind woman brought back to me the memory of my
younger brother. He suffered from a severe, unrelenting bullous
disorder of skin that blinded him and eventually took his life.
After he lost his vision and before he died, he lived by his other
senses in ways that astounded all of us children. He would
recognize and call out by name when one of us tiptoed on the
veranda in front of his room to avoid receiving errands from
him. Senses seem to have a consciousness of their own; they
know how to compensate for loss.

I have written about the cortical monkey for several
years now. All during these years, not once did I see the beast
in the cortical monkey the way I saw him through the blind eyes

of the woman as she disappeared in the snowstorm. My brother and the blind woman saw so much through their blind eyes. We see so little with our seeing eyes.

The American gladiator does things the hardest way. Split ligaments, torn muscles, bruised ego, and all. Winning is not everything for the gladiator. It is the only thing.

Life is tough for the American gladiator. When he is not cringing in cortical clutches, he is bitten by the limbic dog.

****

" .... *a state of body awareness in which the right stroke or the right movement happens by itself, effortlessly, without any interference of the conscious will .... The game plays the game; the poem writes the poem; we can't tell the dancer from the dance .... the doer has wholeheartedly vanished into the deed .... It happens when we trust the intelligence of the universe in the same way that an athlete or a dancer trusts the superior intelligence of the body.*"

Lao-tzu in *Tao Te Ching*
Translated by Steven Mitchell

Chapter 6

Unto the Rising Sun

There is a sculptor in the sky with a gift for every moment. Look up with the language of silence, receive the gift and treasure it.

Life on planet Earth is sustained by a spinning ball of fire — the sun. The sun gives us light and energy. Light and energy bring forth life.

Living things need light to sustain them. Some rare species of fish that live in total darkness deep within the caverns of large caves are an exception.

Tiny buds raise their heads from beneath piles of dirt to seek the light and warmth of the sun. Sunflowers follow the motion of the sun. Little saplings covered by the thick brush of the forest floor lean and bend and twist to peek at the sun. Young leaves on treetops surge high to claim the early rays of the morning sun. Butterflies come to life with the rising sun, and so do woodpeckers. Roosters have different kinds of light sensors; they know when the sun will rise before it actually rises.

The sky reveals. It enlightens. It offers communion. It nourishes. It sustains. It does so at every single moment. Early man knew it. The Egyptians and Sumerians knew it. The men of the Age of Reason knew it. And those who flew up to touch the moon knew it.

On Sunday afternoons I drive to Blairstown for evening office hours. My cortical monkey assists me for part of my journey, but most of the trip finds me fascinated by the sculpture in the sky. The western sun paints the sky in a hundred different colors in a thousand different shades. The underlit clouds have a way of reaching the deepest recesses of human perceptions — and the human soul.

Early man from the Rift Valley in Central Africa gazed at the sun when he was overwhelmed with grief. He did the same when he was happy and wanted to celebrate. When things happened that he didn't understand, he looked up again for answers. There he found his *spirits,* his *gods.* His children, the early Egyptians, had many gods, but the god they revered most was the sun god, Amun-Ra. From him they sought sustenance, and protection from the elements. From the man from Africa, we also inherited our sacred rituals. From him we learned how to begin our fasts before sun rise and break our fasts at the dusk.

There is a gold-colored relief in the tomb of King Ikhnaton of Dynasty XVIII. Ikhnaton is known best for his outspoken challenge to Egyptian polytheism. He declared that the only god was Aton. The gold relief shows the king, his wife Nefertiti, and their two daughters. One of the princesses sounds a sistrum. The king and queen make offerings of flowers to the sun, which hangs above as a sundisk, with the traditional uraeus. It is a precious work of art, stunning in detail and overwhelming in sheer beauty. There is something touching in this relief. A careful look reveals the sun rays turning into little arms as they reach down to make contact with the royal family: God himself reaches down to His people.

The ancient Egyptians had many gods. They worshiped Isiris, Isis and Horus — the father, mother and the son gods.

There was Thoth — a cousin of my cortical monkey and my favorite — the baboon-headed god who invented hieroglyphics, and Anubis, the jackal-headed god who protected the dead from the evil spirits. They had loin-headed gods, cow-headed and snake-headed gods. Egyptians loved to restructure their gods. But there was no god like their sun god, Amun-Ra. At night he traveled below the belly of earth Egypt and emerged from the east in the morning, bringing light, life and love.

From where did the Egyptians inherit their preoccupation with the sun? Their need for some linkage with what must have seemed to them as the center of things in the sky? And their ritual of looking up to the sun for their supreme god? I suppose it was passed down to them from their ancestors from Africa as well. Early man in Africa searched for linkage with something larger than himself. He found that in the sky and in the sun.

Every Sunday, as I drive to my Blairstown office, I see the sky painted crimson, red, pink, purple, silver and gray. The sky changes by the moment. Sun rays turn into little arms that extend down to the creation below. God reaches down to His people. Unkind images of yesterday melt away as do the feared miseries of tomorrow. What permeates the world above and around Interstate 80 is the sunlight, sunlight filtering through the skies in an ever-changing mosaic of light, life and love.

FACING THE RISING SUN

I do my daily limbic rug-running facing east. On the many

occasions when I have experimented with doing the same exercise while facing the west, an interesting phenomenon occurs. When I exercise facing west with closed eyes, I usually find myself facing east at the conclusion of the exercise. Even after a 15 to 25 minute limbic run with closed eyes, this never happens when I run facing east. I open my eyes at the end to find myself facing east just as I did when I started the run. I don't know what the significance of such an observation might be. Did the ancients ever make such an observation? Could such an observation have contributed to their preference for facing east during meditation? I do not know. What I do know is that even in the absence of any scientific evidence supporting the positive effect of facing east while exercising, I recommend it to all my patients.

Historically, there has been an emphasis on facing east for morning meditation and exercise in almost all major cultures. This is a point of considerable interest to me. Is it pure serendipity? What does the east have to do with our mornings anyway? Does it have something to do with the rising sun? Or the electromagnetic field of the planet Earth? Facing the rising sun evidently means our body is aligned with the axis linking the North Pole with the South, the axis of the geomagnetic fields of the planet Earth. A growing body of experimental data indicates that the magnetic field of planet Earth has a profound impact on the biology of all living organisms. Did the ancients know anything about it? If so, how did they?

THE ELEPHANT-HEADED GOD

My friend, Madhava Subbarao, M.D., knows of my interest in the impact of the electromagnetic field of the Earth on human biology. One day he told me about a custom in his native town in India. People there are forbidden from sleeping with their bodies oriented in such a way that their heads point to the north. They can sleep when their heads lie directed to the south or the east. The west is also not considered a safe direction. I asked him why that was so. "Who knows?" He smiled. "As a boy I did that because my grandmother would never let me do otherwise." I asked him if he had any idea as to what the basis for such advice might be. He smiled again. "Listen to the story of Lord Ganesha. My grandmother would tell it to me every time she wanted to make sure I did not sleep with my head pointing to the north.

"Lord Ganesha once stood guard outside the entrance to the pool where his mother, the wife of Lord Shiva, bathed. Lord Shiva came to visit his wife. He was stopped at the entrance by Lord Ganesha. Lord Shiva failed to recognize his son Lord Ganesha, as did Lord Ganesha, his father. Lord Shiva tried to force his way in. Lord Ganesha swore to protect the entrance to the pool with his life. In the battle that followed, Lord Shiva prevailed, decapitating Lord Ganesha.

"When Lord Ganesha's mother learned about the death

of her son by the sword of her husband, she was stricken with grief and cried inconsolably. It was then that she was told how her killed son could be brought back to life. Her husband was to go out in the wilderness and cut off the head of the first animal that slept with his head pointing to the north. That animal was an elephant. Lord Shiva cut off the head of that elephant and put it on top of the neck of the dead body of Lord Ganesha. The dead body of Lord Ganesha stirred and momentarily came alive. To this day, Lord Ganesha carries an elephant head."

Myths fascinate me. Myths are the legacy left to us by the ancients — a true record of how they thought life should be, not necessarily how the life might have actually been for them. The paleontologist ponders the pottery they bequeathed to him to learn how they existed; I reflect on their myths to search for what they might have considered to be the essence of the human condition.

"So! What do you think?" I asked Subbarao.

"So what?" He shrugged his shoulders.

"So tell me, what does the story of Lord Ganesha say to you?"

"I don't know." He shook his head.

"Do you think your folks knew about the electromagnetic fields of Earth?" I pressed him.

"How do I know? I just told you the story my grandmother used to tell me. You are the energy man, you go and figure this one out." Dr. Subbarao flashed one of his disarming smiles.

THE TURTLE AND GEOMAGNETIC ENERGY

Animals travel with biological maps and compasses. They use them to determine their location and to define their direction during their travels. Recent studies clearly show how geomagnetic energy guides some animal species in their migratory patterns.

Florida loggerhead sea turtles have a sophisticated and reliable ability to orient themselves in the ocean. Mitochondrial DNA studies suggest that some turtles literally circle the Atlantic ocean before returning to their native sea off the Florida coast. The results of other studies suggest that sea turtles navigate long distances in their complex migratory patterns by taking cues from the Earth's magnetic fields and the seasonal patterns of ocean waves. (*Scientific American,* 266:100; 1992).

Some other studies show the presence of iron-containing magnetite crystals in some species of bacteria. The bacteria use these crystals as swimming magnetic compass needles that orient them with respect to the Earth's magnetic field. Magnetite has also been found in other animal species such as bees, birds and fish, and appears to allow such animals to navigate by compass direction. Such studies are opening new windows to the world of magnetic fields and their role in biological phenomena. What was seen as metaphysical or paranormal — or simply delusional — can now be clearly understood as physical phenomena.

DO HUMANS HAVE ANY MAGNETIC SENSES?

People have often wondered whether some hitherto un-recognized magnetic sense can explain some human experiences that are generally dismissed as paranormal, and hence scientifically invalid. Physicists have assumed for decades that human beings do not possess any iron-containing magnetic material in their brains. This belief has been used as scientific evidence by some that humans do not possess any magnetic sensitivity. Indeed, this notion has also been used by some in the government and mainstream medicine to deny the presence of any link between weak electromagnetic fields associated with power grids and increased incidence of some types of childhood cancer.

Now comes hard evidence to the contrary. Caltech geobiologist Joseph Kirschvink and colleagues recently discovered crystals of magnetite mineral in human brain cells. Though the concentration of these crystals in the human brain is considerably lower than it is in bees, birds and fish, it is still a significant finding that may hold the key to understanding certain human function in some fields that are often designated as intuitive.

Some known aspects of geomagnetic energy — and some of its biological effects — suggest exercise done while facing the east offers some distinct physiological advantages over exercise done facing the west, however hard scientific proof is not yet forthcoming.

First, electrons from the north pole of a magnet are thought to spin in a counterclockwise direction and generate a positive energy field, while those from the south pole spin clockwise, generating a negative energy field. Second, positive energy excites biological systems, and, when not counterbalanced by equivalent negative energy, leads to a hyper-excited state and ill health. Negative energy — in the context of the Earth's magnetic field — is restorative. Third, all living cells are energy entities, albeit weak ones. In a given magnetic field, the cells "take on" the polarity of that field. For instance, the application of negative energy to a cell causes its negatively charged DNA molecules to spin in a direction that facilitates the entry of oxygen (a paramagnetic phenomenon) into the cell. Fourth, the brain and nervous system appear to have a positive energy drive during the daytime — a state of enhanced excitability that facilitates a day's work. During the night, the polarity of the nervous system seems to change — a change that facilitates a period of diminished excitability and repose.

Now let us consider the possible energy effects of running or doing other types of exercise while facing the east. The right shoulder faces the "negative restorative energy of the South Pole" while the left shoulder faces the "positive excitatory energy of the North Pole." The limbic state may be expected to reverse the polarity of the nervous system, inducing visceral stillness and silence. The right side of the brain (with the probable dominance of the seats of emotions, affections and other limbic qualities) will be more exposed than the left side of the brain to the restorative healthful negative energy of the South Pole. Running while facing the west may be expected to have the opposite effect. Farfetched? Yes! True? Possibly! Will this hypothesis be ever supported by experimental data? Probably!

LORD BRAHMA AND THE SOLAR PLEXUS

The solar plexus, also known as the celiac plexus, is a cluster of nerve cells situated over the spine behind the stomach, liver, pancreas, spleen and the upper bowel. I suppose that early anatomists chose to call it the solar plexus because the nerves of this plexus spread out from the nerve cells like sun rays radiate from the sun. This plexus regulates the principal organs involved in the digestive-absorptive functions of the gut.

I finished writing this chapter on last New Year's Day. As usual I began my morning with a limbic ghoraa run, and within minutes my eyes closed. Sometime during that run, images of the solar plexus and the third chakra emerged, colliding with one another. Later that morning while in the shower I realized that I had failed to make the connection between the solar plexus of nerve cells and fibers and the third chakra, although I had known about both for years. I shook as I saw the eerie possibility of a link between the anatomists' solar plexus and the mythologists' third chakra.

According to the ancient Indian healing philosophy, chakras are energy centers of the human body. The third chakra was sometimes called the Brahma center, a center that held the sum total of all personal as well as universal experiences, a sort of "abdominal brain." In Hindu mythology, Lord Brahma, the creator, dwells in this chakra. I might add here that Lord Vishnu, the preserver, lives in the heart, while the domain of Lord Shiva, the destroyer, is the brain — the residence of my cortical monkey.

Human molecular defenses are plants rooted in the soil of the bowel contents. This simple statement is the synthesis of my studies of the immune system and bowel diseases. As a hospital pathologist, I have examined more than 12,000 bowel and stomach biopsies during the last 25 years. The contents of the bowel, of course, are determined by two sets of elements: 1) what we eat; and 2) what the body organs regulated by the solar plexus do to what we eat. I discuss this subject at length in my monograph *The Altered States of Bowel Ecology and Health Preservation.*

How did it come to pass that the ancients situated the Brahma center, the center of creation at the solar plexus? How did the ancients know that the solar plexus regulated the *epicenter* of human biology? They didn't have microscopes to examine the inside of the gut nor did they have any instruments to analyze what was in the gut. With all our advances in medical science and technology, we are just beginning to recognize the central role of the bowel in health and disease. How did the ancients intuite where the solar plexus was and what it did? Is it sheer serendipity that the biologist situates his epicenter of life in exactly the same place as does the mythologist his center of creation? And the ancients put Lord Shiva, the destroyer, where we locate our cortical monkey? Myths again!

Is it mere folklore that the ancients spoke of the value of facing the rising sun during prayers, meditation and exercise? Or was it a case of enormous intuitive insight? Centuries before we were to learn about electromagnetism and the effects of magnetic fields on biology, the ancients seemed to have known it.

EARLY MORNING MOLECULAR TURMOIL

What time of the day do people experience most molecular turmoil under their skin? What hours of the day do most people suffer heart attacks? What hours of the day do most people develop strokes? Increased stickiness (aggregation) of blood platelets is an important factor of heart attack and stroke. What hours of the day are the blood platelets most sticky and the tone of the arterial walls most pronounced? And what time of the day are the levels of adrenaline and other catecholamines, the aging-oxidant molecules of stress, the highest? Research studies done in different countries point to the same answer: the early morning hours. I cite two studies that address the issue of the occurrence of sudden cardiac deaths, strokes and increased stickiness of platelets during the early morning hours (*Circulation* 75 (1):131; 1987; and (*N Eng J Med* 316:1514; 1987).

On a superficial level, the stress and physical activity

after rising from bed may be expected to cause all this. Right? Not really. This is a common misconception. A visiting lecturer recently spoke at our hospital about circadian rhythm. He was convinced that all these changes occurred as a result of the stress of daytime activities. His advice for avoiding heart attacks and strokes: Stay in bed. A novel approach to preventive medicine!

Regardless of whether or not this lecturer gave his advice in jest, he didn't have his facts straight. I cite below some relevant studies.

.... thus the early morning increase in ST segment depression does not appear to be explained by differences in extrinsic activity and/or stress measured by physical activity score and heart rate response.

Circulation 75 (2):395: 1987.

Translation: There is increased stress on the heart during the early hours of the morning, but it does not appear to be related to the physical activity of getting out of bed and preparing for the day's work. Thus, the heart attacks that occur during the early morning hours cannot be prevented simply by not leaving the bed!

The answer to preventing early morning heart attacks

and stroke is gentle limbic lengthening of muscles, tendons, ligaments and other types of connective tissues followed by slow and sustained limbic exercise at the beginning of the day, and a visceral stillness during the day. This is *true* prevention.

Each day signals a new beginning. A new awareness of man's relationship with his world and the light, life and love that surrounds him. A renewed link with the larger *presence* that surrounds him.

CIRCADIAN RHYTHMS AND THE PINEAL BODY

The ancients knew and respected the circadian rhythms in biology. They recognized many physiological phenomena related to these rhythms, and most of their rituals coincided with them. Because we physicians have been trained to reject everything outside the domain of our drugs and surgical scalpels, we have been quick to dismiss all aspects of circadian rhythms and their impact on human biology. This is beginning to change. Some oncologists — albeit in hushed tones — now tell me that certain chemotherapy drugs may be less poisonous to their patients if administered with consideration to certain aspects of circadian rhythms.

The pineal body is a small pea-sized organ in the brain that secretes some hormones including melatonin. The pineal body depends on natural light for its function. Abnormal levels of melatonin, and most likely some other related pineal body hormones, cause severe mood and mentation disorders. Indeed, melatonin has been reported to be of clinical value in alleviating symptoms caused by jet lag. Circadian rhythms affect heart, brain and hormonal functions. In fact, studies show that body organs suffer as a result of natural light deprivation.

The relationship between natural light and health has been empirically recognized since humans began to record history. In recent decades, this subject has been studied extensively in animal experiments. When animals are deprived of natural light, they become lethargic and listless, and lose their fur and weight. With extended light deprivation, animals become sterile and develop abnormal patterns of bone development. Development of full-blown clinical picture of SAD has not been reported in animals when they are deprived of natural light. How would animals express their sadness in ways that can be double-blinded and crossed-over by our researchers in medicine? I wonder.

Is it any wonder that I am partial to the morning and to the eastern sky when I exercise. The morning sun creates the best in limbic lights and the best in limbic images. I write more about this subject later in this chapter.

CHILDREN OF FLUORESCENT LIGHT

Natural light is one of the primal needs of man. It is the irony of our time that Americans — who take pride in living in the richest and most powerful country in the history of man —

are so widely deprived of natural light. The human species is being pushed more and more into artificial fluorescent light, and farther and farther away from natural light. Morning was a precious time for our ancestors. It still is for all of us.

Natural light sustains life and restores health, and the lack of natural light plays many roles in the cause of mood disorders. People who suffer from depression know their vulnerability is increased on overcast days. These problems are most pronounced in sufferers of seasonal affective disorder (SAD).

Access to natural light is being denied to an ever-growing number of our children at home and at school. When they become irritable, confused or inattentive, we readily diagnose hyperactivity syndrome or attention deficit disorder and promptly write out prescriptions for Ritalin or related drugs for discipline. Up to 6% of all children in the public schools of the county of Baltimore have been reported to be on drugs for discipline (JAMA 260:2256;1988). I discuss the relationship of nutritional and environmental factors to attention deficit disorder in *The Butterfly and Life Span Nutrition.*

Exposure to natural sunlight has been drastically reduced for many children due to changing sleep patterns. Increasingly, small children are kept awake for long hours by late night TV. They are taught in classrooms with fluorescent lights. It seems to me that natural light deprivation is at the root of many of our schoolchildren's mood and mentation problems, though I am not aware of any extended scientific studies of this subject.

I'LL ALWAYS LIVE ON THE WATER

Sometime ago, my brother-in-law, Hanif Bajwa, moved to a high-rise apartment with an open view of Miami harbor and some islands in the distance. With considerable joy, he spoke of the healing quality of the water. He spoke about how therapeutic the water view had been for his stress level. "I find looking at the water so comforting," he concluded, "that I have decided to always live on the water."

Who wouldn't? Almost everyone I know would live on the water only if he could. The problem, of course, is that most people cannot. If people cannot live on water, can they live on the sky instead? The sky has an enormous comforting and healing power. The sky can be everyone's water. Most people go through life never knowing that. The sculpture in the sky is infinitely more varied, more enriching and more comforting than the sculpture on the water. The tragedy is that we blind ourselves to this ever-present, ever-enriching source of beauty, comfort, and yes, spirituality.

OPEN UP THE SKY TO YOURSELF

The American gladiator *does* things differently. If he

were ever to be convinced that the sun might indeed have anything to offer him, he would want to climb up to the sun and demand it. The gladiator is not alone in this. Most gurus in the advice industry think the same way. They regularly give recipes to their flock for opening the sky, as if the sky exists only to be opened up by their clever words.

Can anyone really open the sky to himself? I do not really know but it does seem very unlikely to me. What I do know is that every person can learn to open *herself or himself* to the sky. There *is* a difference between the two. How can we open ourselves to the sky?

There is no need to seek beauty in the sky, only that we relinquish our notions of what beauty is and what it isn't.

LIMBIC LIGHTS

Limbic rug-running with closed eyes brings forth a limbic play of unique colors, shades and lights. These shades and lights appear and disappear randomly as I inevitably pass from limbic openness to cortical thoughts and back to limbic silence again. Following are some patterns of colors, shades and lights I often see with my limbic eyes during my ghoraa run.

THE LIMBIC GRAY

Overcast days usually bring forth a diffuse gray openness (the limbic gray) that surrounds me. Bursts of light then rupture the gray, scattering and illuminating its parts with numerous shades of gray, silver, blue and white. The parts of the gray coalesce to form new unbroken sheets of gray. And then the cycle repeats. The diffuse gray breaks up into floating masses of gray that turn and twist and bump into each other before coming together again to make up the diffuse, unbroken gray.

On some days I sense the gray openness around me during the early minutes of my run even when the sky is clear and light blue. As minutes roll by and I slide more deeply into limbic awareness, the limbic openness that surrounds me changes its colors to gray-white, silver, blue and then white. It seems to me that gray is the color of the cortical monkey; it persists in its various shades, pulling us back to cortical thinking, until the monkey is banished.

THE LIMBIC GOLD

The limbic gold is the gold, crimson or yellow-red color

that fills the space before the closed eyes facing the sun on clear, cloudless days. For the beginner, it largely represents bright sunlight filtering through closed eyelids. Indeed, a clear image of the sun as a bright yellow disk frequently hangs somewhere in such fields of color. These colors are often broken by waves of lighter colors or streaks of darker colors as the eyelids flicker. As I am carried further into limbic openness, the direct light filtering through my closed eyelids becomes an unending display of motion and change. The limbic gold turns into a dazzling array of colors that blend, emerge and blend again into an ever-changing kaleidoscope of colors.

THE LIMBIC SILVER

For the beginner, limbic exercise done on days when the sky is open but has sparse clouds will usually bring forth a silvery openness (the limbic silver) before his closed eyes. As in the case of limbic gray, this silver openness will appear and disappear as he or she shifts from cortical clutter to limbic listening and back to cortical clutter again. Also, as in the case of limbic gray, a person with a strong capacity for limbic perceptions will soon see other shapes of limbic openness even when the sky is cloudy.

THE LIMBIC BLUE

Contrary to what one may expect, limbic blue is a late event during progress with limbic exercise. Limbic openness shifts from one shape to another, and from one color to another — except to a deep blue — even when the sky is azure blue. When the limbic blue does takes form, the person is usually transported into the deepest and the widest of all openness.

The limbic blue represents a deep limbic state. As I begin my limbic run, blue speckling on a sheet of gray often appears before my closed eyes on overcast days. In time, blue speckles coalesce and become small blue patches. On days that I slide very deeply into a limbic state, the blue eventually spreads and the gray dissolves, leaving behind a clear deep blue that one sees in the desert on a clear sunny day.

THE RAIN FOREST EFFECT

Just before my eyes spontaneously close during limbic exercise, my upper eyelids usually begin to droop. The effects of light filtering through partially closed eyelids usually allow an escape to limbic openness. Often, sunrays passing through a shielded window or through tree trunks create visual effects reminiscent of the rain forest. Sometimes the light is soft and filters as if through the mist of a rain forest, at other times it arrives in sharply defined rays as if the light of a blazing sun were cutting narrow slits through the dense tree trunks. At yet other times, it resembles a continuous stream of raindrops falling like translucent pearls. These effects vary by place, time of the day and weather, but they have one thing in common: They kill all impulses to engage in the *percent* games forced upon us by exercise experts.

THE GHORAA RHYTHM

There are two essential elements of limbic exercise: the ghoraa rhythm and limbic openness.

As previously stated, ghoraa rhythm refers to a natural, effortless exercise rhythm. Non-analytical and non-judgmental, it is a pattern of exercise in which the legs find their own rhythm, the head bobs rhythmically and swings with gentle to and fro motions, the shoulders drop a little with each step, the flesh in the loin shifts a little with each forward thrust of the hands, the torso floats along effortlessly and the whole body moves at its *own* speed. There is no sense of competition, no definition of goals, no hunger for scores. It is the rhythm with which ghoraas pull tongas over long runs in Pakistan. It is the rhythm with which horses pull carts and buggies in this country when they are *allowed* to *find their own rhythm*.

THE LIMBIC DOG AND THE KHOPPA EFFECT

The Khoppa Effect is the ablation of all visual distractions. The Khoppa Effect, described earlier in this chapter, is essential to success in limbic exercise.

I know many people who become very uncomfortable when they close their eyes. Sometimes my patients show palpable anxiety as they close their eyes during autoregulation training. It is quite apparent to me that they live in a state of molecular overdrive. A young man literally froze as he closed his eyes. I asked him to open his eyes and tell me if he knew why that happened.

"Dr. Ali, you have no idea how much energy I spend in just existing. There is nothing left for me to do other things," he replied.

Such individuals live with the internal chemistry of the fourth of July — with molecular fireworks that feed upon each other. They frantically expend their total energy to preserve an external calm — a desperate attempt to maintain outside control. The darkness of closed eyes becomes insufferable.

The limbic dog is not into biting. Not out of revenge, he bites out of utter confusion, a total lack of control over his innate reflexes. He has been defenseless for so long. A little kindness, a small display of affection, a soft touch is all that is needed to throw him off balance. People who suffer from extreme stress, acute anxiety, panic reactions and depression need to understand why their limbic dog bites. It is only through such understanding that they have any chance of true relief.

It is possible to meditate and do autoregulation with open eyes. Indeed, I urge all my patients to learn to do "minute-reg" (minute-reg is autoregulation done for a minute or so at a time). During initial training in limbic breathing, however, the Khoppa Effect is difficult to achieve without closing the eyes. For safety, while training, eyes should be closed during limbic exercise only when the body is supported by hands as with an exercise cycle or a treadmill. People with ear or balance disorders and those with a history of dizziness must not attempt to close their eyes during exercise unless supported. Most other individuals can, with training and practice, learn to close their eyes without losing balance.

Limbic breathing during limbic exercise is very valuable in this stage of progress. I have described limbic breathing in *The Cortical Monkey and Limbic Breathing*. I include a brief outline of this mode of breathing in the chapter The Limbic Pacing And Limbic Exercise. Lactic acid is one of the principal fatigue molecules. It also plays an important role in anxiety and panic attacks. Limbic breathing significantly lowers the blood levels of lactic acid and other fatigue and stress molecules. Limbic breathing also decreases the blood levels of adrenaline and its cousin, stress molecules. By these and several other effects, limbic breathing done during limbic exercise increases the stamina of tissues for exercise. When the benefits of limbic breathing combine with those of banishing both cortical clutter and the cortical monkey, the full impact of limbic exercise becomes evident.

LIMBIC IMAGES

A limbic image is a limbic experience. In *The Cortical Monkey and Healing,* I define the terms cortical images and limbic images. A cortical image is created by the thinking mind. There is no element of *unexpectedness* in it. The limbic image, however, is completely unexpected. There is nothing *expected* about it. It comes to us as a total surprise. Usually the first response to a limbic image is, "Oh, what was that?" This cortical thought, of course, immediately dissipates the limbic image. With time, a person doing limbic exercises (or autoregulation) *allows* himself to sustain such images. The limbic images form and dissolve as he slips into and out of the limbic state.

LIMBIC OPENNESS

During limbic running, limbic openness often becomes a huge canvas upon which limbic images appear and disappear. I do not try to analyze them (that, of course, would immediately end the image). I never interpret them. Frequently, an image that follows some days later seems to link up with an earlier image, and the two images lead to yet another image. I believe such linked images represent a "limbic intelligence system," the purpose of which is to enlighten us and raise our consciousness far beyond our daily mundane activities. This system works well for me. Indeed, the most important parts of this book took form during my limbic runs.

Here are some specific examples of limbic images that I have seen.

In limbic openness, I see a tree branch. The branch changes its form and looks like a staghorn. Momentarily, a head of a stag appears next to the staghorn, and then a second staghorn takes shape. The two staghorns are then transformed into the spread out wings of an eagle. The wings enlarge and widen till they reach the limits of perceivable openness. Then the image dissolves completely and there is nothing but limbic light — a wide, wide limbic openness.

On another occasion, I see a small metal hook. The hook enlarges and changes into an Imam's Mehrab (the archlike structure under which a Muslim Mullah stands to lead his followers in prayer). Then the Mehrab widens and its pillars spread out. The arch grows in size, becomes circular and dissipates into a huge ball of light. The ball of light dissolves into an openness.

One day during my morning run, my thoughts drifted to a study in which some oral surgeons had wired the jaws of their obese patients so that they could not eat solid foods. Next, they put them on liquid diets. For these oral surgeons, of course, this was *research*. The innocent and gullible victims of this research lost weight which they promptly — and utterly predictably — regained after their jaws were released. I felt a surging anger at these "researchers." "Idiots!" I muttered under my lips. Then I realized what I was doing and made a deliberate effort to banish those thoughts.

I soon escaped into limbic openness and became conscious of a comforting blue-gray openness all around me. Suddenly I felt my neck sheared away from its base above my shoulders and transfixed a few inches laterally to the right. Although quite uncomfortable, the sensation of carrying a severely mal-aligned neck did not frighten me. My patients had often related variations to me. I call this phenomenon *cortical de-braking* and discuss it in my book *The Limbic Dog and Directed Pulses.* I resisted the temptation to open my eyes and terminate this disturbing image, however, it eventually dissolved. Sometime later I wondered if this image had anything to do with my anger at the surgeons who had wired the jaws of their unsuspecting victims.

One day I saw the limbic light in the form of a crescent. A vertical band of light appeared to give it the semblance of a cross. Next, the cross assumed a starlike configuration, the sharp angles softened and a large circle of light took form. The circle of light finally dissolved into limbic openness. This sequence of images may mean different things to different people, but for me it simply happened that way. I have no interpretive comments here.

Sometime ago, I tried to compare the effects of limbic running with the Khoppa Effect to that of jogging. I jogged on a beach track looking at the ocean waves breaking out on the white sand and then I ran limbically at the same place with eyes closed.

NEWPORT BEACH AND LIMBIC OPENNESS

On clear summer mornings in Newport, the air by the ocean is usually crisp and fresh, the breeze exhilarating. The view of the glistening ocean water is mystifying. Running becomes limbic even without trying. I ran looking at the ocean for a while and then with my eyes almost closed, barely perceiving the running track before me. When the track was clear even for a few yards, and my half-closed eyes seemed to want to shut, I let them do so. I discovered something interesting. As much as the ocean water was soothing to the eyes, limbic openness seen through closed eyes was more captivating. Each time I gave my eyes the option, they chose to exclude the ocean view, exercising a clear preference for limbic openness.

DOG DAY MORNINGS

Mornings should be celebrated. In the preceding chapter, I give my reasons for my viewpoint. I recognize that many people who may want to put my suggestions to test will counter two problems: the problem of the cortical monkey and the equally vexing problem of the bites of the limbic dog. Morning is a cortical time for most of us — a time for thinking about a dog day ahead, a time to brace for the punishments that the dog day will put out for us. We rush to our coffee and doughnuts.

For many of us, when we do escape the cortical traps in the morning, we fall prey to the bites of the limbic dog. The connective tissue does not yield, nor do the stiff muscles let go. The torso sends out distress signals, the limbs limp along in pain. The bites of the limbic dog become sharper as the cortical monkey continues to pile up yet more punishment.

GO FOR THE MORNINGS, DAYS WILL FOLLOW

The morning for me is a time for gratitude, a deep sense of gratitude for being alive, for being able to spring out of bed. I know many people who cannot do this. It is a time for looking up at the sculpture of the great sculptor in the sky. It is a time for the language of silence.

For many years when I was a disease doctor, my mornings escaped me. There used to be this great rush of preparing for the chores of the day. My mornings do not escape me now. The problems of the day get addressed pretty well *when* they appear. Certainly there is no energy wasted on excelling in things that do not need to be done in the first place.

There are many mornings when my watch advises me to miss my morning. I have to leave early for a conference at the hospital or a medical staff meeting. (God knows there are too many of them.) Sometimes I am travelling and my watch tells me the morning belongs to the travel schedule. My watch does not govern me in the morning anymore. How did that happen?

Exercise is boring. Everyone knows that. What moron really enjoys endless running at a time when a warm bed is the place to be? What runner's high or endorphin surge can match the joy of lazy, lingering moments in a warm bed? I know it is true because, like most people, I had my flings with morning runs.

I have come to know that perception of energy in tissues is not compatible with unyielding connective tissue and pulled muscles. Nor is the capacity for looking up at the sky with the language of silence congruous with tightness in the chest or knots in the stomach. Indeed, these are mutually exclusive. I have also come to know that for me limbic lengthening is a necessary prelude to communion with the sky. Finally, I have come to know that what may seem improbable to many is a simple occurrence for me: Limbic impulses take over my mornings, and I simply follow wherever they choose to take me.

Water has a special sustaining value in the morning. I take about 16 ounces of water with my supplements after limbic lengthening of my neck and back tissues. I follow this with another eight ounces of vegetable juice with one and half tablespoons of a partially digested protein (peptide and proteins) formulation. I walk out onto the covered patio with a skylight. My limbs want to move and I simply follow them. My torso floats very much like the torso of the ghoraa I used to watch on my trips to Kirto.

I know I am not into exercise. I am into my mornings, and my mornings are most giving when I yield to them, for 20 to 30 minutes or more. My mornings give me my days. I remember my days were different when my mornings were not there to give them to me.

So I tell my patients to take the lead of their mornings. The days, I know, will take care of themselves.

A NEW DAY, A NEW AWARENESS

Morning is the best time for limbic exercise.

In my view, whatever one does for exercise later in the day, he must have a *daily* morning time of exercise and silence, even if this period can be only for a few minutes. Also, this time must include a few moments of initial neck, back and limb stretching, and some forehead and temple message. I have several sound reasons for this recommendation.

First,

morning sets the tone for the day. We usually wake up

with the cortical monkey. This monkey, of course, loves to recycle misery of our yesterdays. When that doesn't sustain him, he pre-cycles the feared future misery of our tomorrows. All of us need to unclutter our minds in the morning. There is no better way of doing that than limbic exercise.

Second,

morning offers several physical and mechanical advantages over all other times for limbic exercises. Morning is the best time to relieve the strain on muscles, tendons, ligaments and other connective tissue that results from one's sleeping posture. Reverse isometric exercises for neck and low back muscles are essential preventive measures against chronic neck and backaches.

Third,

morning is the best time to obtain a state of slight overhydration for the rest of the day. Most of us stay in a state of dehydration when not making a conscious effort to drink fluids. I discuss this subject at length in *The Butterfly and Life Span Nutrition.* From personal observations I know that my general level of energy and sense of well-being is profoundly effected by my state of hydration. During the first one hour of the morning before I leave for the hospital, I drink about 36 hours of fluids — half as plain water with my nutrient supplements and half with a peptide and protein drink mixed with

vegetable juice. Five days a week, this carries me
through to lunch time at about 1 PM. Coffee or tea are
not a part of my morning. Without this much fluid, I
sense a need for coffee the way I used to before I
changed from being a disease-doctor to a physician
devoted to health and preventive medicine.

Fourth,

most people can control their schedule best in the
morning. All that is required is rising a little earlier (and
going to sleep a little earlier, a small price to pay to start
a new day right.

Fifth,

The early morning hours are a time of high molecular
turmoil. This time, I discuss earlier in this chapter,
carries some well-recognized hazards for people with
heart and vascular disorders. Limbic lengthening followed
by slow, sustained exercise offers considerable protection
from these risks.

Sixth,

and most importantly from my personal perspective, the
morning is the best time for perceiving the energy of the
native human condition. It is a time for limbic openness
through limbic exercise. It is a time for silence. It is a

time for higher states of consciousness, a time for *being*. It is a time for seeking a link between the gentle guiding energy within us and the gentle guiding energy around us — the energy of that larger *presence* that surrounds each one of us at all times.

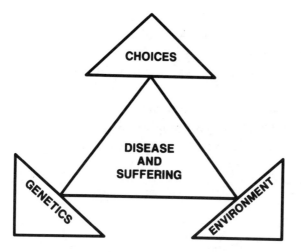

Theray khaillayan nouh luggay purr
Rubb lubbaiy khitthay ohh chullhay
Na randha ooh khittaban which naah
biabaan which

Rubb they dhou kurr
Ik uchhi chuth thay utthey
Doujhaa chup dil they which

✸✸✸✸✸✸✸✸✸✸✸✸

Your imagination takes to wings
You search for Him in vain
He lives not in books, nor in wilderness

God lives in two temples
One high above the heights of heavens
The other deep in the depth of a silent heart

Chapter 7

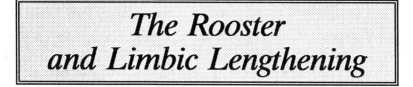

The Rooster
and Limbic Lengthening

Roosters flutter their wings to announce their morning. Canaries flap their feathers before they fly off their nests. Dogs stretch before they take their first steps. So do cats. We humans wake up to our coffee and begin to recycle the misery of our yesterdays and map out the feared future sufferings of our tomorrows.

A rooster crowing in the early hours of the morning brings me the essence of the morning. It is a time for a new beginning, a renewal of a sort. A time for gratitude for being alive, a time for a silent celebration of life. For the Chinese, a rooster crows to dispel evil spirits that might descend upon people as they sleep during the night.

Sometimes my thoughts wander and I reflect on the essence of the morning, and how mornings have changed from the way they used to be for most people — even as recently as a century ago. Then I think of how little they have changed in the animal kingdom. Nature has its own sense of order. It has its own notions of life, harmony and balance. It has given animals a clear sense, what we call intuition, for living their lives with vigor and health — that is until we arrived on the scene and began to mindlessly and relentlessly destroy their habitat.

How did that happen? I suppose we can say animals are still *connected* to nature. They still take their cues from it. They respond to it. So do plants and trees. Indeed, so do individual body organs, tissues and cells. As I write this, I see the issue of *Science* I received yesterday. It includes a fascinating article about circadian rhythm.

We now report that isolated cultured neurones (nerve cells) from the molluskan retina (inner eye membrane) exhibit circadian rhythms.

Science 259:239; 1993 (Parenthesis added)

There is an irony here. Physicians who practice drug medicine dismiss all notions of health and disease except those that fit into the prevailing *standards* of medical care. They deride the very notion that circadian rhythms have any relevance to their clinical practice. Biologists continue to extend their observations about nature's working. They document with careful studies how single cells respond to cues from nature and *autoregulate.*

So how did it happen? Why are animals and plants still *connected* to nature? How did we humans get so disconnected? Animals have spontaneity of motion; we have little, if any, of that left in us. I suppose one answer is: Animals still do what nature wove into their DNA sequences; we humans are punished by our own schemes. Animals live by instincts, we live by the dictates of others. Do people have any instincts? If not, why not? Why would nature deny us what it considers so essential for animals? And plants, I might add. If nature did give us instincts but we don't have them now, what happened to them?

ROOSTER'S LENGTHENING
AND THE GLADIATOR'S STRETCHING

Limbic lengthening in my autoregulation terminology is gentle, *sustained lengthening of the connective tissue* in the ligaments, tendons, sheaths of connective tissue that surround muscle fibers and cells in other body organs. The term muscle stretching is commonly used for stretching the muscles with various rapid, jerky motions. *While stretching of the muscles cells (fibers) has its value, it is not nearly as important as lengthening of the connective tissue.* This is an essential point in the physiology of fitness.

Muscle stretching, as it is commonly practiced, is stressing the muscles with abrupt, jerky movements. We Americans like vigorous bone-cracking stretching. That way we can tell we actually did something. Is that necessary?

At the fall 1991 meeting of the American College of Advancement in Medicine in Reno, Nevada, I served as the program chairman for one session. After the first two papers were finished, I decided to give the audience a one-minute break. On an impulse, I led the audience through some reverse isometric exercise (described later in this chapter) to loosen up the tissues in the neck and dissipate any restrictions in the muscles of the back and neck that often develop during long periods of sitting in one posture in medical conferences. The exercise took about two minutes. After I finished the exercise, I asked the physician group how useful they might have found the exercise. My colleagues responded generously with applause. I resumed the program and called upon the next speaker.

Someone approached me after the program was over, and said, "Dr. Ali, there is something very important you missed." He shook his head with thinly disguised disappointment and continued, "When you teach anyone such exercises, you must be very careful. You must warn them not to apply more than sixty percent of the maximum force." I thanked him for his advice and promised him that I will try to remember that. He walked away, still shaking his head.

GOD SAVE OUR PERCENTAGE POINTS

And God bless our experts who swear by their percentage points — and live by them. Our exercise experts are infatuated with numbers. Sixty percent of the maximum force! How do I find out what that 60% is? I wondered. How can I find 60% of *any* force unless I know what 100% of that force is? And how do I find out what that 100% force might be for any of my patients? By forcefully bending his neck until it breaks? How do I find what 60% of that force might be for my own neck? By having someone bend my neck with progressive force until it breaks?

I wondered if this "expert" knew what 60% of his maximum force might be. *I do thank him, however, for he has provided me with one of the clearest examples of what "cortical monkeying" is all about.*

CONNECTING WITH THE CONNECTIVE TISSUE

How does the rooster know how hard he needs to flutter his wings in the morning? What are the rooster's percentage points for his flutter motion? How does a cat know how much she should lengthen her limbs? What are the cat's percentage points for lengthening of her limb tissues? How does a dog know how long he has to stretch his torso? What are the percentage points for his tensile strength? How does a canary know how hard and how long she needs to flap her wings before she flies off her nest in the morning?

In limbic exercise, of course, the answer to this is very simple: We should put as much tension on the connective tissue in our ligaments, tendons and muscle sheaths as these tissues will naturally accept — without provoking any protest from them. Translation: We need to learn how to perceive energy of tissues and how to be guided by it. From a practical standpoint, there is an important issue: How much pressure does the connective tissue take before it rebels? As connective tissue regains its natural suppleness and resilience, the muscle fibers will take their cues and grant us a spontaneous fluidity of motion. I wonder if my expert, in his worship of his Gods of percentage points ever reflects upon such matters.

A clear understanding of what the connective tissue in the body is, how it works, and how it gets injured is of paramount importance in any fitness program. The connective tissue connects all tissues — and no tissue can maintain its structure or function without the support provided by this tissue. Muscular fitness cannot be achieved without fitness of the connective tissue. Nor is it possible to attain cardiovascular fitness without supple and resilient connective tissue. Fat-burning enzymes cannot be up-regulated without a supportive connective tissue. The same holds for other aspects of metabolism and the function of other body organs. If there is parallel to spiritual connectedness in the domain of physical fitness, it is "connective tissue connectedness." Connective tissue literally serves the tissues as their anchor. Without this connectedness, tissues are nothing more than jumbled masses of tissue soup, unable to breathe, unable to move, unable to respond to work demands — and unable to live. It is evident that the connective tissue must be protected from injury in all fitness programs. Injury to connective tissue is the principal reason most people who undertake ambitious exercise abandon their exercise. Injuries to the connective tissue call to a halt all fitness activities.

Below I discuss some essential aspects of the anatomy (structure), physiology (function), pathology (injury and degenerations) of connective tissue as a prelude to specific recommendations for limbic lengthening of connective tissue before and after exercise. Painful trigger points caused by torn and ill-repaired connective tissue in ligaments and tendons — usually in close vicinity of joints — are common reasons why most people are forced to discontinue their fitness programs. In the chapter Limbic Exercises for Specific Disorders, I include an outline of the treatment of myofascial trigger points with proliferative therapy using 50% glucose solution, a method that I have found to be extremely useful for facilitating the healing process.

STRUCTURAL ASPECTS OF CONNECTIVE TISSUE

The cells in the human body may be seen as bricks; the connective tissue makes up the mortar that holds individual cells together. It is present in various proportions in all tissues, some tissue contain more of it than others. The cells of connective tissue — fibroblasts and mesenchymal cells — play the central role in tissue healing. These cells provide the scaffold for repair of other tissues. In wound healing, these cells provide the glue, much like cement is used to hold together individual bricks when a brick wall is broken.

CONNECTIVE TISSUE IS A THINKING TISSUE

The connective tissue is a living tissue. It has sensors for sensing the state of tissues in its environment. It takes an accurate measure of demands put upon it — and it responds accordingly. Not only can the cells of connective tissue make functional adjustments, they can adapt their structure to meet the changing demands. For example, such cells can turn into osteoblasts and form bone, become chondroblasts and lay down cartilage, or assume the role of cells that form new blood vessels to bring in more blood and nutrients. When the tissues are damaged beyond repair, the connective tissue cells synthesize collagen, the dense tissue of scar.

Some tissues are made up almost exclusively of connective tissue. Examples of such tissue are ligaments, tendons and aponeurotic sheaths — thick bands of very strong, resilient structures that connect muscle fibers with bones. Connective tissue is the protective tissue for muscle, for cartilage that covers the bone surfaces in joints, and for other soft tissues in and around joints.

GOLGI TENDON ORGANS: THE SENTINELS

Golgi tendon organs (GTOs) are tiny structures located at the junctions between the tendons and muscles. These organs house pressure and stretch sensors. When tendons and muscles are subjected to sustained stress, the GTOs sense the force and duration of stretch and pass this information to muscle cells that respond to these signals by elongating — a process that in reality represents absence of muscle cell contraction. This is a physiological process, the benefits of which are readily felt by everyone, though often at a subliminal level. Indeed, when we sit on a chair for a while and then shift our position, it is in response to the impulses generated in GTOs. The result is limbic lengthening of our muscles and connective tissue and an increase in tissue flexibility.

FUNCTIONAL ASPECTS OF CONNECTIVE TISSUE

The connective tissue of the body is resilient tissue capable of withstanding enormous distortion. It has a high degree of elasticity and returns rapidly to its original length after being lengthened. Muscle cells are motor cells of the body. They serve this function by their contractile properties. This is generally well understood. What is not commonly appreciated by people who do not exercise regularly is that this cell has a unique ability to lengthen greatly when it is required to do so. Athletes know this, and use this aspect of muscle physiology as the centerpiece of their conditioning programs.

LIMBIC RANGE OF MOTION

A full range of motion of the various joints in the body is of central importance to fitness and health. The range of motion — flexibility of tendons, ligaments, other types of connective tissue and muscles that govern motion at specific joints — is essential for spontaneity and fluidity of movement. It is determined by the type and level of activity performed, presence or absence of structural musculoskeletal restrictions, temperature of the tissues and the age and gender. Increasing tissue temperature increases the range of motion and cold temperature decreases it. Women usually have a larger range of motion.

Deprivation causes distortions, and to paraphrase Disraeli, absolute deprivation of the connective tissue causes absolute distortions in its function.

This must be recognized as the key element in all programs for fitness for a life span. Children prevent deprivation — and distortions in the function and the structure of the connective tissue in ways that are similar to those of the rooster. Adults and the elderly develop such distortions through the deprivation of non-use. The full range of motion cannot be maintained except through *daily* limbic lengthening of the connective tissue. The common wisdom received from our exercise experts that exercise done three or four days a week can support muscular and cardiovascular fitness — as they are so fond of calling it — is sheer nonsense.

WHAT IS LIMBIC LENGTHENING?

Limbic lengthening is elongation of connective tissue and muscle fibers that occurs when these tissues yield with a natural spontaneity of motion. The tissues *do* yield spontaneously when they are allowed to do what comes naturally and effortlessly to them. Abrupt and jerky movements that pass for muscle stretching among our fitness gladiators are mere devices of the cortical monkey. Such movements only annoy tissues and provoke further resistance from them.

A common practice in spas and gymnasiums is to practice muscle stretching in groups. I do not recommend this practice. How can one person be guided by the tissue energy of another? How can one person know the limits of the tissues of another person? How far are the tissues *willing* to yield? No one can answer this question for another person. Group stretching almost always becomes a competitive pursuit; everyone steals glances at others. Everyone takes a measure of everyone else. The trainers usually are skillful at hiding their own cramps and stiffness from their trainees. Their time to attend to sore and rebellious tissues begins after the trainees have returned home with their stiff and sore tissues. The American gladiator thrives.

Limbic lengthening increases tissue flexibility. Specifically, in the context of joint motion, flexibility refers to the range of motion of a joint or a series of joints. From an exercise standpoint, it is more useful to consider individual joints or a series of joints as functional units that integrate the functions of muscles, tendons, ligaments, and even bones that participate in joint motion. Limbic lengthening prevents injuries such as pulled muscles, sprained ligaments, tendon tears and specific injuries such as shin splints and Achilles tendinitis.

THE BULL AND MILO OF CROTONA

In ancient Greece, Milo of Crotona fell in love with a newborn calf. He played with him and lifted him every day. With passing months, the calf grew stronger and heavier. Milo's arms also grew stronger and heavier as he continued to lift the growing calf every day. Several more months passed. The calf grew into a young bull. Milo kept up his practice of lifting the young bull, and so maintained his ability to lift the bull. Some more time passed. The young bull grew into a fully grown, massive bull. And yet, Milo continued to lift his bull every day at sunrise. The news of Milo's feat spread far and wide. People traveled from long distances to see if Milo could really lift his massive bull all by himself. Milo surprised everyone.

Myths are cryptic notes bequeathed to us by those who went before us — a common heritage of a sort for Man. Often I do not fully understand them. When I do, they have a guiding influence on me. The ancient Greeks were astute observers of the human condition. The story of Milo is an eloquent tribute to their understanding of the physiology of human fitness. In antiquity, they understood intuitively what our exercise experts still do not — with all their reams of computer printouts: that the central issue in fitness is the *consistency and naturalness* of activity. I think of Milo every time I hear some exercise expert talk about 70% of maximal aerobic capacity. Or when they advise their students to exercise three or four days a week.

The ancient Greeks knew something about the resilience of the connective tissue. And of the suppleness of muscles. They knew some things about the rigidity of the connective tissue and of the spasticity of muscles that comes with the punishment of neglect and disuse. I sometimes wonder how different myths would have been if the common folks in ancient times had begun their mornings with coffee and doughnuts. How would have the ancient myth-makers seen the punishment of pulse rate percentage points? How would they have written their myths? What would be the myths about people who drop dead on pavements in desperate pursuit of assigned percent points?

PATHOLOGIC ASPECTS OF CONNECTIVE TISSUE

Over the years, I have cared for a large number of patients with limb injuries suffered in sports and accidents. Among them, injuries to ligaments, tendons and other types of connective tissue were very common, and those of muscles quite uncommon. Muscle injuries, in general, heal rapidly; those of the connective tissue, much more slowly. One obvious reason for this is that the muscle tissue is very rich in blood supply while the connective tissue is poorly supplied with blood. In chronic pain syndromes of the neck, back and limbs, the painful trigger points are situated in the connective tissue much more frequently than they are located in the muscles. Furthermore, the clinical benefits are far greater when the focus in treatment is on the injured connective tissue rather than the muscle. I discuss this subject in greater detail in the chapter Limbic Exercise for specific health disorders.

RECONSTRUCTIVE ASPECTS OF CONNECTIVE TISSUE

My viewpoint that the connective tissue is the tissue of central importance in any exercise program has been fully validated for me by own clinical experience with the diagnosis and treatment of myofascial trigger points with reconstructive proliferative therapy. As I look back, I recall very few times when I found it necessary to treat painful trigger points located within the muscles themselves. The vast majority of these trigger points that I have personally treated were clearly situated within the ligaments, tendons and aponeurotic sheaths. In my clinical experience, the most effective therapy for these trigger points is prolotherapy — a form of therapy in which 50% glucose solution is injected into the damaged connective tissue with equal parts of xylocaine. I discuss this subject at length in the chapter Limbic Exercise for Specific Health Disorders.

I MUST BE KIND TO MY CONNECTIVE TISSUE

Unstretched ligaments and tendons are uneasy ligaments and tendons. They brood and bruise easily. Withdrawn and sullen, un-lengthened connective tissue shuns participation, much like a shy child backs off when other children on the field coax him to join them, even though he yearns to be among them. Un-lengthened muscles are unhappy muscles — tentative and resistent, willing to participate in the motion but uncertain of themselves. Lengthened muscles are kind muscles.

I sense the response from my own connective tissue and muscles fully each morning during my own moments of limbic lengthening before I start my limbic running. My muscles are somewhat tentative as I get out of the bed. They do respond to me but not with a great degree of enthusiasm. This, of course, changes rapidly as I do my regular neck, shoulder, back, hamstring and calf stretches.

Limbic lengthening has a way of turning into stretching, stretching into slow motion of running in place, running in place into jumping jacks, and then back into slow motion running. This is how I often settle into a limbic run. Every now and then I find myself breaking into a sprint and limbs settle back into a deeply restorative limbic state.

I must be kind to my connective tissue so my connective

tissue can be kind to me.

LIMBIC LENGTHENING IS NOT THE SAME THING AS WARMING UP

Warm-up refers to physical activity that raises the body temperature, and hence the temperature of the connective tissue, muscles and other body tissues. Life in essence, I wrote earlier, is enzyme function. Enzymes are what separate living things from inanimate objects. Temperature is one of the basic factors that control enzyme function. It follows that even slight reductions in body temperature can adversely affect enzyme performance. This, I might add parenthetically, is one of the principal reasons why people with underactive thyroid gland function have low body temperatures, and suffer from low energy and sluggish metabolism.

Warm-up activities are of two broad categories: 1) Related warm-up that is undertaken primarily to raise the tissue temperature in specific groups of tissues such as slow cycling with short sprints before a cycle race; and 2) General (unrelated) warm-up in which the activity undertaken is different from the actual exercise of interest. The related warm-up is of interest primarily to competition athletes and has little relevance to limbic lengthening and limbic exercise. The important point of considerable practical value in this context is this: It is important to undertake some form of slow, sustained activity to raise the temperature of tissues before doing vigorous stretching. I know many people who strain their ligaments and tendons from abrupt and forceful stretching movements and have to relinquish their exercise program altogether.

"Whatever warm-up you choose, it should be intense enough."

So reads a line written by one of the well-known exercise experts. The cortical monkey is alive and well. So is the American gladiator. Intensity is the only game in town. It is the buzz word of our time. Intensity at work. Intensity at play. Intensity for winning. And winning — we learned our lesson well — is not everything. It is the only thing.

Our exercise experts are into intensity. Their motto is: "No pain, no gain." How does it hurt our tissues? How much? How do tissues protest when they are driven with intensity? Such concerns are of significance for our experts. As for limbic lengthening, advice like the one quoted above is utterly irrelevant.

THE HEART, LUNG AND MUSCLES
COME OF AGE IN 1990

I am as much amused by the "experts" of fitness as I am

by the "experts" of nutrition.

In 1978, the experts at the American College of Sports Medicine published "The Recommended Quantity and Quality of Exercise for Development and Maintaining Fitness in Healthy Adults." In that year, cardiorespiratory and muscular fitness was not deemed worthy of inclusion in the title of their recommendations. In 1990, these very experts at the College made a landmark discovery: The heart, lung and muscles are important for fitness programs. Twelve years after the first guidelines, the experts at the College — in some moment of great enlightenment —   chose   to   add   the   words "Cardiorespiratory and Muscular" before the word "Fitness" to the title of their recommendations.

But wait! That's the way science moves, silly, I can hear the experts say with scorn. How would a mere pathologist understand the subtleties of our specialty? The experts at the College   are   likely   to   exclaim   in   scorn.   The   1978 recommendations were for maintaining health and those of 1990 are for training for fitness.

"Strength training of a moderate intensity, sufficient to develop and maintain fat-free weight should be an integral part of an adult fitness program," the experts at the College declare in their 1990 pronouncement. So strength training was not essential in 1978 but was so in 1990.

The experts at the American College of Sports Medicine are sharp with their numbers. They are up on their statistics and down on common sense. They pronounce — with great authority that can only come from a sure sense of self-righteousness — that the *right* frequency of exercise is three to five days a week.

Translation: There is not much point in daily exercise more often than three times a week. These experts caution us that gains in maximum oxygen uptake tends to plateau after three days a week. They emphatically peg the intensity of exercise at 60 to 90 percent of the maximum heart rate. Sixty percent, they insist, is the minimum threshold for improvement in maximal capacity. These experts are fascinating people. They thrive on what they regard are subtleties of exercise — too subtle to be comprehended by common folks.

That brings me to the important subject of scientific non-progress.

SCIENTIFIC NON-PROGRESS

We Americans, I wrote in *The Cortical Monkey and Healing*, are a numerical people. We love numbers. We cherish them. We live by them. We are sustained by them. When deprived of them, we crave them. We seek safety in numbers. Without our numerical crutches, we are vulnerable. Modern medicine is a numbers game. Numbers tell us how to label our pain. Numbers define the magnitude of our suffering. Numbers give us our diagnostic labels. Numbers give us our treatment strategies. We conduct research with numbers. To generate our research, we happily blind ourselves. Dissatisfied with simple blinding, we invent methods to *double-blind* ourselves. When double-blinding does not give us sufficient gratification, we devise yet more clever schemes for confounding the issues — we develop methods of *cross-over* for our numbers so that no one can ever use common sense in looking at the data.

Next time you hear an exercise expert from the College make his pronouncements, think of the philosophy and the principles and practice of fitness of the Assyrians, the early Egyptians, the ancient Greeks, the American Indians and the African tribal message carriers. Then think of all the patients with heart disease who suffer chest pain and suffer from heart attacks while they desperately try to reach the *numbers* prescribed by the exercise experts of the College. Or those who suffer from painful arthritis and are advised to take painkillers before they exercise. Or those who are sentenced to three to five periods of punishment on concrete pavements, burning their brains out in their quest to reach the pulse and breathing numbers assigned to them by our exercise experts. Or lower the blood cholesterol levels by a few points. What passes for *science* in the fitness industry, in most instances, is nothing but the marketing goals of men of money of the fitness industry. Common sense is so uncommon in health matters these days.

LIMBIC POSTURE

Function of tissues cannot be understood without the study of their structure. It is a sad state of affairs when a surgeon limits his knowledge of the human anatomy to only that which serves him in the use of his scalpel. It is equally tragic when an internist is interested in structure only to an extent that is necessary for performing his procedures. We physicians almost universally ignore the essential knowledge of human posture and the adverse effects of abnormal posture, first on our musculoskeletal system and later on other visceral organs. The way we walk can either keep our body muscles and ligaments free, limp and loose, or throw them into a frenzy of misdirected boluses of electromagnetic energy.

Gravity is an inexorable force. It puts upon us a pressure of about 34 pounds per square inch of our tissues. It is gravity which causes our body tissues to sag down or fall out with age.

During early embryonic development, human organs develop in segments. That means that all the body organs developing from one particular embryonic segment will be supplied by the set of nerves which develops from that segment. This explains why people who suffer from myocardial infarction (heart attack) frequently develop pain in the left shoulder or left arm. The heart sitting in the center but leaning to the left side of the chest develops from the same embryonic segment as does the skin of the left arm and the left shoulder. Similarly, people who suffer from gall bladder disease experience pain in the right scapular region (upper part of the posterior chest wall). This phenomenon is designated as referred pain, and the principle behind it is called Hilton's Law.

The critical importance of this phenomenon should be readily apparent to us. What hurts muscles in a segment will also hurt other body organs in that segment. How does that happen?

An old man who is a smoker of many years suffers from

a cold and develops a persistent cough. He is involved in a car accident and develops a whiplash injury to his neck. His neck and shoulder muscles are in an intense spasm. Days pass without any relief. His cough and chest pain get worse, he develops progressive musculoskeletal restrictions, his breathing becomes increasingly labored, the inflammation in his lungs caused by the viral infection becomes more intense, he comes down with pneumonia and needs a respirator for survival.

An over-dramatization? Visit the intensive care unit of your hospital on any day, listen carefully to patients with heart and lung disorders, and you will gain some insight into the workings of the human frame.

A second case is a young man who walks with his head thrust three inches in front of his shoulders. He considers this his "normal" walk. He often suffers from headaches. His physician tells him he has tension headaches which come from "nerves." He is advised to take aspirin for his headaches. Some months go by. One day his *normal* daily headache is not relieved with aspirin. On TV, his favorite celebrity urges him to try the celebrity's favorite double-strength brand for which the celebrity is paid handsomely.

What do these two men have in common? The body tissues of both suffer from repeated boluses of misdirected energy. The old man is likely to see how the spasm in his neck muscles drove him to the respirator. There is little chance that the young man will see how each step taken with an improper posture (with his head thrust three inches in front of his shoulders) puts stress on his neck muscles. It can be seen as a mini-whiplash with each step. His head hurts because the muscles hurt a thousand times each day. Little does his physician realize the irony in his diagnosis of stress headache caused by weak nerves. How can he? He never recognizes the maladaptive posture in the first place.

What is limbic posture? It is the posture which our body assumes when we let it. It is a posture free of contortions, free of muscle tension, free of pain. It is a posture with fluidity in tissues and spontaneity in motion. How can we tell? By limbic listening. By trying different postures and listening to tissues locked in those postures.

Stand sideways before a mirror and observe.
Are your ankle joints exactly below your knee joints?
Are your knee joints exactly below your hip joints?
Are your hip joints exactly below your shoulder joints?
Are your shoulder joints exactly below your ears? (This last step requires either two mirrors with angles or the help of a friend)

Why is it desirable to stand erect like that? Because this is the line of gravity along the coronal (front to rear) plane of the body.

Now stand erect, feet pulled together, facing the mirror. Observe.

Are your two ears at the same level?
Are your two shoulders at the same level?
Are your two hips at the same level?
Are your two knees at the same level?

This gives us a view of our posture along the sagittal (side to side) plane of the body. Why is this important? So that the pull of gravity is sustained by our bodies in the way Nature meant it to be.

Observing the level of the hip joints usually requires an extra step. Put your hands on your abdomen with fingers touching the bellybutton. Move your hands downward and outward until they meet the two bony points above the hip joints (anterior superior iliac spine). Bend forward and roll the fingers below these bony prominences and straighten up. You will clearly see whether or not the two bones are at the same level.

Now try to stand erect, correcting the abnormalities of posture you may have recognized. If this limbic posture causes discomfort, we know the work we have to do. We never force tissues. Autoregulation is about listening to tissues. It is not about ordering them around. In advanced cases, we may need professional help to dissolve the myofascial trigger points which cause us to lose our natural limbic posture. Usually, however, simple awareness of a problem in posture will effortlessly bring about the change through limbic exercise.

LIMBIC WALKING

Limbic walking is walking in the limbic posture.
The body posture is erect and limp and loose.
The head does not swing side to side or front to back.
The neck carries the head as if the two were but one

supple piece.
The shoulders retain their normal alignment.

The spine moves with forward flexion and backward extension. There is no rotary motion (rotation causes torque, and torque causes muscle stress, micro-trauma, spasm, pain and abnormal posture).

The arms swing back and forth in a forward and backward arc to dissipate the momentum. They do not cross in front of the abdomen, swing behind the hips, rotate inward, or rotate outward. The legs move in three distinct motions: a heel kick, a midstance, a forward propulsion.

I reiterate that self-observations are necessary for understanding. Cortical, competitive attempts to correct the "abnormal biomechanics" overnight with exercise or with manipulations has little chance of long-term success. I return to limbic perceptions of tissue energy. Body tissues know how to respond if only we let their energy guide us. Once we let ourselves be guided by the tissues, we cannot be "un-guided. Once we know something, we cannot un-know it again. Cortical compulsions cannot molest the tissues anymore.

LIMBIC RUNNING POSTURE

I define limbic running posture as a running posture in

which *all* body tissues move with ease, naturally, effortlessly and rhythmically. There is no muscular or ligamentous contortion.

I described earlier in this chapter the physiologic alignment of the torso and limbs and the neck and head into a natural posture. The essential point I wish to make here is this: *There should be no attempt to change our usual posture overnight in order to do limbic exercise.* Yes, it is our ultimate objective to return to the natural posture, but attempts to regain it should be *limbic*, gradual and sustained.

Following are some illustrations of the way people run.

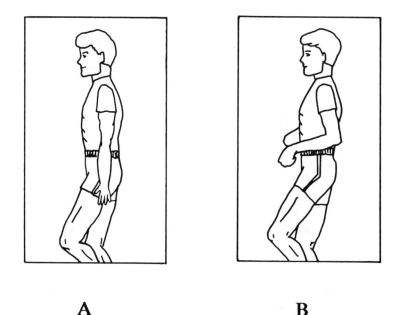

A   **B**

The runner in illustration A shown above keeps his arms

rigid and close to his sides. This posture robs him of natural fluidity of motion in his arms and eventually puts stress on him. In illustration B, his left shoulder is pushed out backward, his left elbow is sharply flexed, and his neck is stretched forward. This posture again robs the runner of a natural running posture, and will cause dysfunctions of connective tissue and muscles, and, with time, internal viscera.

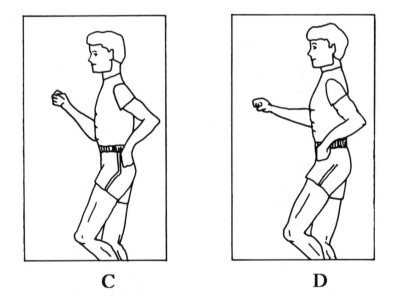

C   D

The runner in illustration C has a better running posture that those in illustration A and B. Still, his left elbow is sharply angulated and swings it too far back with his step, putting unhealthy stress on his left arm, shoulder and neck muscles. His right arm swings far too high, again putting unhealthy stress on his right arm, shoulder and neck muscles. The runner in illustration D has a natural posture for effortless limbic running. This posture is most compatible with limbic running for long periods of time without wearing out any specific groups of muscles and ligaments.

It is important to note that necessary changes in the running posture should be *allowed* to happen. Cortical attempts to quickly straighten the posture overnight or in some days or weeks are likely to add to the problems of poor posture. Limbic exercise is about taking counsel from the tissues and not from the cortical monkey.

REVERSE LIMBIC LENGTHENING

"Reverse limbic lengthening" — reverse LL — is a set of physical steps that allow gentle, sustained lengthening of the connective tissue and muscle fibers. Reverse LL free musculo-skeletal restrictions by putting gentle tension on the connective tissue and muscle fibers in directions opposite to the ones in which they are normally stretched. The essential point in reverse LL is this: We should *never* use a degree of force which makes us uncomfortable. On the following pages are five steps for specific reverse LL for the neck that are very beneficial for people with chronic pain and stiffness in the neck. Before you try these five steps, move your neck gently in a circle and feel the presence or absence of any muscle stiffness or pain. Now follow the five steps of reverse LL.

First Step

Rub the neck and shoulder muscles between your two palms to loosen them and warm them up for one or two minutes. Next do a temple message with a gentle, rolling motion of your palms placed on your temples as shown in the illustration.

Second Step

Turn your neck to the right as far as it will go without causing any discomfort. Put your left hand firmly on your left temple as shown on the next page (A). Push your neck firmly against the left hand. There should be no actual movement in the neck, the push of the neck should be balanced by the push of the hand. Count to ten and let go.

Third Step

Turn your neck to the left as far as it will go. Put your right hand on your right temple as shown on the next page, and follow the same instructions for the left as for the right (B).

Fourth Step

Bend your neck forward, as far as it will go without causing discomfort. Put your two hands on the back of the head as shown above. Push your head up against the two hands firmly but without discomfort. There should be no actual movement of the neck (C). Count to ten and let go.

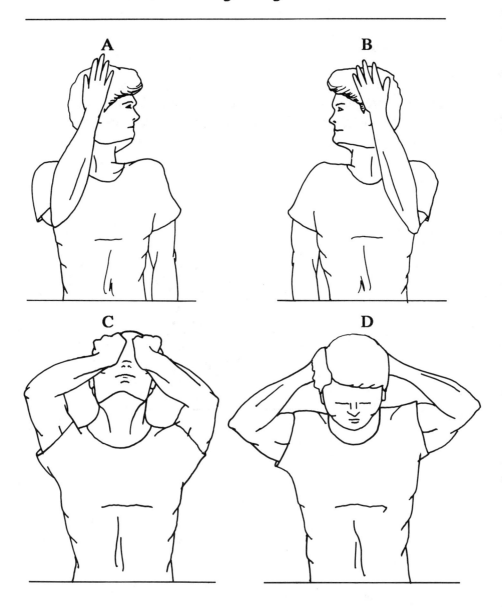

Fifth Step

Extend (bend backward) your neck. Put your two hands on your forehead as shown in the preceding diagram, and follow the same instructions for bending your neck backward as for bending your neck forward.

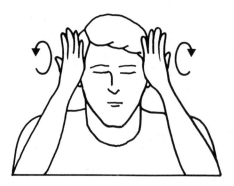

Sixth Step

Move your neck in gentle circles as shown above and see

how much freer your neck now is compared with the same movements before doing the preceding five steps.

Reverse LL for specific muscles of the shoulder, back, thighs and legs can be developed using the principle of reverse isometrics. If necessary, a professional may be consulted for learning reverse LL for different parts of the body.

Reverse LL, performed several times during the day while doing one's work, must be considered essential parts of a structured program for reversing catabolic maladaptation.

I begin my day with reverse LL for the neck muscles and ligaments each morning before I leave my bed. It takes only a few minutes. Next I do leg and thigh stretches. Then I proceed to muscles and ligaments in my back (using the principle of reverse LL). I do my reverse LL for the abdominal muscles as many times during the day as possible, usually a few times each hour. Earlier, during my training period, I had to give myself reminders. Now it is not necessary. Often, the reverse LL *come* to me spontaneously and without any conscious effort on my part.

LIMBIC LENGTHENING OF MUSCLES

Limbic lengthening of the connective tissue and muscle fibers is essential for success in limbic exercise.

Effective limbic lengthening must include all major

muscle groups of the back, thighs and legs. The principle of limbic lengthening is the same regardless of what body tissues are in play: Muscles and ligaments are stretched in a gentle and sustained fashion. Again, we *never* put pressure on ligaments and muscles to a degree which makes us uncomfortable. Following are four types of reverse LL that I highly recommend before doing the ghoraa run or other forms of limbic exercise.

The first exercise illustrated below seeks gentle limbic lengthening of ligaments, tendons and muscles of the back and the calf. The arrows indicate the locations of gentle and progressive tension in the first step (A). To reiterate, the tension must be gentle in the beginning, sustained and progressive in degree, and should last for one or two minutes. In the second step, the direction of the gentle lengthening stresses on the back muscles changes as shown in (B).

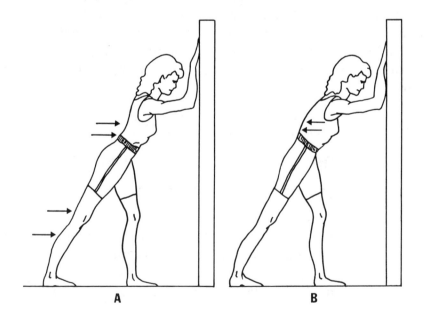

A   B

In the third step (C), gentle, sustained lengthening stresses are applied to a large number of muscles and ligaments in the thigh and leg, and the muscles of back when the individual leans forward to touch the wall (not shown).

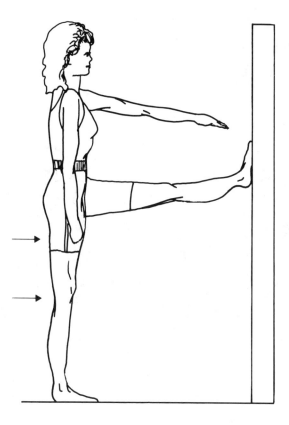

In the fourth (D) and fifth steps (E), gentle and sustained lengthening stresses are put on the thigh, abdominal, shoulder, neck and back muscles. This exercise is more

demanding than those illustrated above. I do this exercise after
I have finished my limbic run, when my muscles and ligaments
have been loosened and invigorated with limbic exercise.

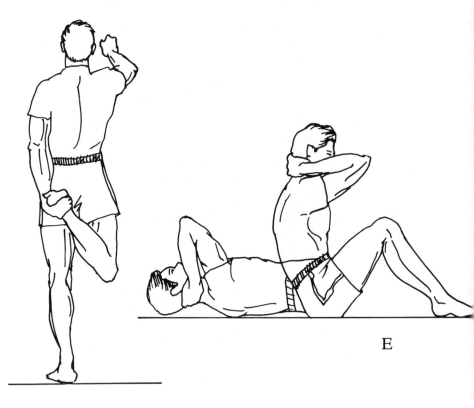

E

D

Some other variants of the same basic exercise are shown below.

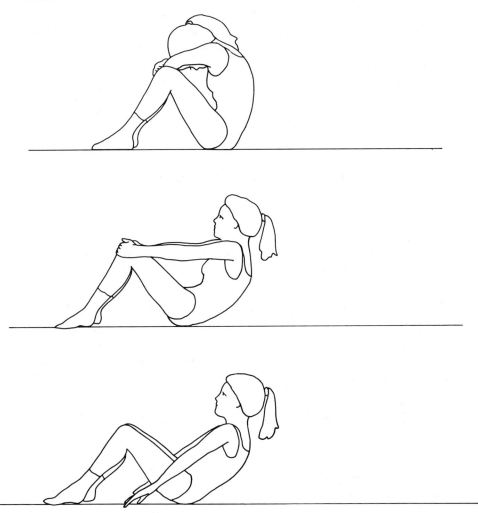

Office work puts physical and mental stresses on the muscles of the neck, shoulders and back. Such stresses can be easily dissipated by simple exercise steps done while sitting on the work chair. If colleagues are amused by the sights of such exercise, I suggest a response that entirely consists of a non-committal smile. Discussions about such matters, we remember, are cortical devices, and distract from the desired limbic effects.

LIMBIC LENGTHENING ON A CHAIR

I illustrate below some simple steps for limbic lengthening of the tissues of neck, torso and limbs while at work. These simple steps, repeated for a few brief moments three or four times during the day, will do more than anything I know to keep the connective tissue supple and resilient, and minimize the possibility of injury. The only "equipment" required for these exercises is a secretary's chair, or for that matter any other type of chair without arms.

Limbic Lengthening of Neck, Shoulders and Back Tissues.

Two simple but highly effective exercise steps are illustrated in the diagrams on the next page.

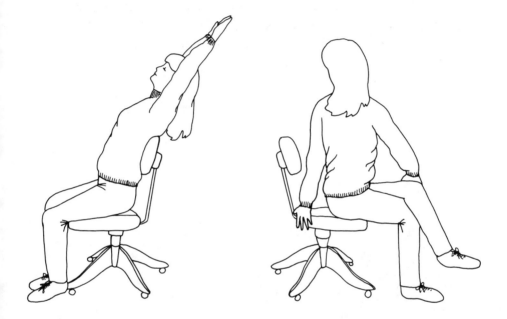

Limbic Lengthening of Thighs

Some additional, simple lengthening steps appropriate at work are shown below. These steps dissipate the rigidity that often develops in the connective tissue, muscles and other tissues of thigh, leg and back at work.

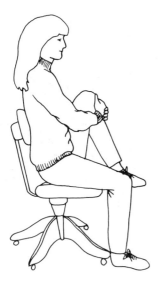 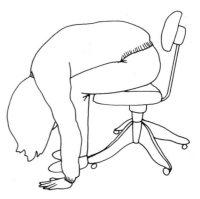

I strongly recommend frequent use of the two simple lengthening steps shown below and on the following page.

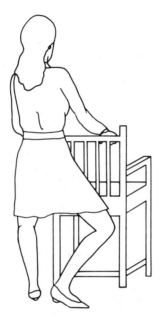

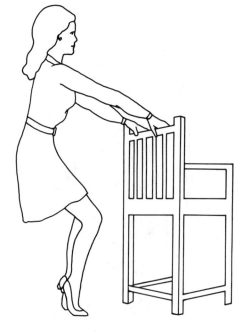

POST-EXERCISE LENGTHENING

Limbic lengthening after limbic exercise is just as important as it is before it. Exercise coaches often recommend that post-exercise stretching should be more intense and performed for a longer period of time than pre-exercise stretching. The main reason, they assert, is that this is necessary to prevent injury to tissues that may occur due to abrupt changes in the muscle activity. This is not necessary in limbic exercise. The reason for this is obvious. In limbic exercise, we are guided by the tissue energy.

In limbic exercise, the cortical monkey cannot molest limbic tissues.

We do not allow our thinking mind to put demands on these tissues. There is no potential here for tissue injury inflicted by our cortical compulsions. Since the mind is not allowed to molest the tissues in the first place, there is no need for prolonged post-exercise lengthening. Slow and sustained lengthening of tissues for a few brief moments is enough.

If a man does not keep pace with his companion, perhaps it is because he hears a different drummer. Let him step to the music which he hears, however measured or far away.

Henry David Thoreau

Chapter 8

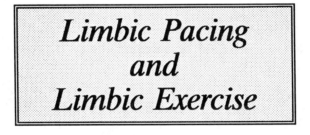

Limbic Pacing
and
Limbic Exercise

Walking, the Natural Way to Up-Regulate Fat-Burning Enzymes

Motion is an essential attribute of life. Since humankind moved from scuttering around on all fours to walking on two legs, it has wandered around, usually without wondering about the nature nor the effects of walking. It has walked for its daily chores. It has walked for a living. It often walked long distances in a native state, limbically — without knowing that walking was beneficial. Walking has been a part of its day. Men and women have walked to be with company, and they have walked to be away from company.

Walking has been good for humankind. Movement is necessary for optimal metabolism and to meet the energy demands of life. Walking calls for no specific goals. It requires no equipment. Any place is the right place for it. Any time is the right time.

The notion of walking for exercise is a recent invention, a creation of the cortical monkey. The cortical monkey, I wrote earlier, is destined to connive and scheme. He cannot exist in limbic openness. He simply cannot *be*.

Walking offers all the molecular metabolic advantages I discuss in the preceding chapters. If we simply allow our limbs to lead us, we will walk — simply, naturally, effortlessly and limbically. If we choose to let our walking experts decide how and when and for what periods of time we will walk, there will be problems.

The American gladiator turns simple, natural walking into a task — a skill that must be vigorously pursued and mastered, with those "whooshy, cushy" walking shoes, head gear and spandex, and with score cards, daily logs, time charts and the reprimands that delinquency inevitably brings.

HOW SHOULD I WALK?

Beginners frequently ask three questions about walking:

How should I walk?
How fast should I walk?
How long should I walk?

The answers to these questions in our language are simple.

How should I walk?
Limbically.

How fast should I walk?
At a limbic speed.

How long should I walk?
For limbic distances.

What kind of answers are those? You ask. Before I explain my answers, let me give the answers our walking experts are likely to give.

The walking expert will answer the first question by saying, "Walk heel-and-toe." He will answer the second question by saying, "Walk briskly enough to raise your pulse rate to seventy percent of the maximum expected rate for your age." Next, he might give you a chart that tells you what the maximum pulse rate for your age should be. He will answer the third question by saying, "You should walk two to four miles every other day." Finally, he will define some goals and set you up with some daily logs, score cards, a timer and some tests.

Now I return to my answers. Limbic walking means when we walk, we simply walk. We do not sit in judgment of how we walk. It is true that heel-and-toe walking is desirable for long walks. Toe-walking and flat-footed walking increase the strain on the leg and foot muscles. But this should not be an issue as we begin walking. Toe-walking and flat-footed walking are problems of nonwalkers. Walkers soon *limbically* fall into the right pattern of walking. If we didn't know that such things as toe-walking and flat-footed walking exist, now we do.

The second question of how fast one should walk is equally trivial. Walking limbically means walking by taking the lead of the legs. It is not walking under the command of the thinking head. There is no demand put upon the legs to perform to any standards set by clever thoughts. We walk without any preconceived ideas. Walking briskly is more effective for up-regulation of fat-burning enzymes than slow walking. Now what is walking *briskly*? Evidently, what is very slow walking for one person is brisk walking for another. How do we know if we are walking *briskly enough*? The answer is by taking the lead of our limbs — listening limbically. If we choose to listen to our legs, they will let us know whether brisk is brisk enough. Our legs will also let us know when to change the degree of briskness as we continue limbic walking and become physically better conditioned.

Counting is a cortical activity. Some exercise programs require that the walker stop at the end of the walk and count his pulse, and do so *immediately* lest there be a slight slowing of the heart rate before he counts. And what, I wonder, will happen if he did start the count after a few moments and the heart rate slowed a bit by that time? Some walking experts do not just stop at that. They want us to go all the way. They want the works. They want us not only to count our pulse rates but also our breathing rates. Then there are those who must offer the rewards as soon as the walk finishes. They develop ingenious scoring systems. When you finish the walk, they admonish us, you must keep an accurate record of your pulse and breathing rates and report to them. They will then analyze our score cards. Nothing for the poor performers, rewards for the high performers. How many of these good boys and girls will go home after their exercises, their raised blood pressure still high, their stomach ulcer still burning? Our exercise experts do not concern themselves with such questions.

As for the third question — how long to walk — the experts come again with their formulas and computations. If we let them, they will even wire us to their electronic gadgets and produce computer bar graphs and pie charts. They will furnish us with numbers that we do not need — and that our cortical monkey thrives upon as it pushes our blood pressure up and pours strong acid on our stomach lining to give us gastritis or ulcers.

Remember, our legs and feet know far more than our minds ever will. Here is a practical suggestion. Next time you run, listen to your legs. When they tell you to stop, stop running and walk. Watch what happens. They will ask you to start running after a while. As days and weeks go by, our legs and feet and arms and torso warm up to us. They will ask us to do what is right for us. There is no right way and there is no wrong way. There is no cortical greed. Just limbic gratitude.

In limbic walking, as in limbic breathing, sometimes the limbic dog bites. When the tissues have been ignored for too long, they may not warm up to us on such short notice. In such times, we need fortitude. The limbic dog, I wrote earlier, is not into biting. When it bites, it bites out of confusion, not vengeance.

LIMBIC PACING

In limbic pacing, our body tissues have the freedom to set the of our exercise. Limbic pacing offers far superior healthful effects than any other "expert" advice. Once again, limbic exercise is intended to attain and maintain the optimal catabolic set point for life span weight. It is not intended for a physiologic advantage over an opponent in a competitive sport. Going limbic in competition sports to cancel out all cortical activity, eliminate stress and seek limbic openness is a different issue altogether.

Limbic exercise, in essence, is done for the same reasons one does limbic breathing, i.e., to obliterate the cortical devices and to still the mind. It lowers the blood lactic acid level and offers us all the molecular and cellular
benefits that result from the limbic state. For effective stress control we need to understand stress pathophysiology. We need to know from where the stress is coming, how much stress we are under, and how we can bring about internal physiologic changes to dissipate the stress molecules. However, when we actually breathe limbically, we couldn't care less for those aspects of stress physiology and stress pathology. We know that all cortical activity is inconsistent with limbic breathing. It is the same with limbic running. We need to know the physiology of running. And yes, we must also know the pathology of running. But when we run limbically, all this is meaningless. Cortical analysis of the process of running negates limbic running. We can run cortically or we can run limbically, but we cannot do both.

LIMBIC EXERCISE FOR THE BEGINNER

Physical conditioning takes time. Also, it takes time to learn how to let the body tissues lead. There are some essential elements that a beginner must address as he follows this path.

1. Safety and Avoidance of Tissue Injury

SAFETY FIRST

Safety first. I described in the chapter The American Gladiator how I regularly see my physician colleagues injure their backs, knees, ankles and other body parts during exercise. Avoiding injury during exercise is not simply a matter of technique and of cortical vigilance. Indeed, that, in my experience, substantially increases the possibility of tissue injury. True safety in exercise comes from following our spontaneous impulses — from taking limbic leads from our limbs. Tissues do not respect the diplomas of our exercise experts and fitness trainers. (Training for competition athletics, I repeat, is a different matter and requires specific goal-oriented training.)

It is very easy for the beginner to sprain his ankles and hurt his legs as he starts an exercise program. This, of course, is the principal reason many people discontinue exercise. Such physical setbacks are less discouraging than the setbacks of deflated egos and bruised spirits. The discouragement that comes from injured tissues is nowhere near as disillusioning as the loss of hope. If someone has allowed himself to become a couch potato, he must not attempt to become physically fit and conditioned for exercise over a weekend or during a one-week fitness camp.

PHYSICIAN REVIEW OF HEALTH STATUS

I cannot overstate the case for a clinical evaluation of one's general health by a physician before embarking upon an exercise program. Exceptions to this rule are children and young adults.

There can be some extreme hazards in exercise for the beginner. In the next chapter, I relate the story of one of the pediatricians on our hospital staff who died suddenly of irregular heart rhythm within days of starting a program of running. Such horror stories are not rare. Others who need close medical supervision for exercise are those who suffer from chronic degenerative disorders.

EXERCISE ATTIRE AND SHOES

There is only one issue here: The attire should be comfortable and should offer adequate protection from the elements. The same holds true for shoes. I described earlier how I run limbically every day at home on a covered patio that gives me fresh air and yet protects me from rain, snow or the freezing winds in the dead of the winter. I run on a three foot by three foot thick rug. Exercise attire is not important for me. I do not wear any exercise shoes. During the winter months, I simply dress warm, warm enough so that the cold air does not stress my tissues before limbic lengthening and limbic running can warm them to a degree that the ambient air does not offend them, even on the coldest of cold days. Simplicity paves the way for a limbic experience.

For those who run on sidewalks or even on running tracks, the choice of shoes is quite important. Well-built and sturdy shoes go a long way in stabilizing ankles and providing support for feet and ankles and preventing injury to tissues. No shoes, however, can prevent injury to tissues that are poorly conditioned and are being driven hard by the misguided attempts to lower blood cholesterol levels or prevent heart attacks. When we walk or run to meet some predefined goals, every single moment of such exercise can be — and often is — punishment for the tissues. As far as I know, cells and tissues only respond to their inner cues and do not much care for those cushy shoes that boast 33% more air or other similar great inventions in exercise gear.

The limbic dog often bites the beginner. Such limbic bites are not cruel tricks of the limbic dog. If the tissues have been neglected for a long time, they may not warm up to us just because we need them on short order. Our tissues do not share our sense of urgency when one day we discover we have heart disease or hypertension and embark upon some great fitness program. The bites of the limbic dog, I wrote earlier, always cease with time. I discuss this subject further in the chapter Limbic Exercises for Specific Disorders.

LIMBIC LENGTHENING
AND REVERSE LL

Limbic lengthening of connective tissue and muscles by putting gentle, sustained tension on them is essential for freeing musculoskeletal structures before exercise. Reverse LL do the same for connective tissue and muscle fibers that are not lengthened by ordinary exercises. I discuss these two important subjects at length in the preceding chapter. The only comment that I repeat here is that exercise that is not preceded by these simple steps is very likely to lead to injured tendons, ligaments and muscles, and to broken promises.

CHOICE OF EXERCISES

What types of exercises can be done well *limbically*? Walking, running, rope jumping, cycling and swimming are all good exercises. The key elements in all these exercises are *continuity* in exercise and opening ourselves to that native state that brings forth the limbic openness. Exercise done with equipment such as treadmills, row boats, mechanical track machines, and others that allow slow, sustained physical activity offer similar physiologic advantages. I know of many people who do go *limbic* while doing such exercises. Some other types of exercises that are popular with exercise experts are pure cortical devices. They are contraptions that our experts invent to turn us into mindless robots. In the chapter, The American Gladiator, I referred to an ugly device called the swimming machine by its inventor. Such devices offer little except insults to our common sense.

Tennis, racquetball, golf, basketball, football, baseball, softball, weight lifting and other similar exercises are good exercises with many physical, emotional and mental health benefits. However, these are stop-and-go types of exercises that frequently involve competitive efforts, and so do not qualify as suitable choices for someone wishing to do exercise limbically.

A comment about aerobic exercises with popular videotapes: These exercises are okay for the beginner, but by definition, these cannot be limbic exercises. Indeed, the cortical monkey rides high when we are really "into" the technique of exercise. Still, video aerobics are good in the sense that any exercise is better than no exercise. A move into limbic exercise is far easier when we are familiar with exercise.

Treadmill walking and treadmill running can be limbic exercises to a degree. The treadmill speed can be controlled and necessary adjustments made. Walking or running may be slow or brisk according to the demands of the tissues. It is easy to stop and start again. With minimal practice, one can learn to safely do these exercises with eyes closed (three-quarters closed or completely closed). Some of my patients find it easy to combine various methods of autoregulation with simple acts of treadmill walking or running.

A necessary element in any type of exercise is to increase duration. Years of inactivity rob us of spontaneity of motion in our joints, muscles, ligaments and tendons. Herculean efforts to rid ourselves of musculoskeletal restrictions so caused are destined to result in failure. Limbic listening to injured tissues may seem like too abstract an idea to be of any practical value. With regular limbic exercise, this *abstract* idea becomes a nonabstract reality.

The concept of rotation, which is essential to my management of food allergies, is also applicable to the efforts for increasing stamina. Specifically, I advise my patients to select a number of exercises that suit them. For instance one may rotate the following: very slow walking, brisk walking, slow treadmill walking, fast treadmill walking, rug running, rope jumping and jumping jacks. The trainee moves from one exercise to another just as soon as his body parts want him to stop the first exercise. Anybody who has ever tried this knows that changing the type of exercise usually is the best protection from the natural urge to stop running altogether. To reiterate, the key element here is listening to the body tissues and abiding by their wishes.

WEIGHT-SUPPORTED AND WEIGHT-BEARING EXERCISES

This is an important issue for people in a poor state of

physical fitness due to age, infirmity or simple inactivity.

Exercise requires *continuity* to be effective in up-regulating fat-burning enzymes by enlarging the number of mitochondria, enhancing enzymatic efficiency and increasing the rate of fat catabolism. Continuity in exercise requires physical stamina. It is a mistake to try to build physical stamina in a hurry. Such attempts only give us aching muscles, sore joints, sprained connective tissue and broken hopes.

Exercise with a stationary exercise cycle is probably the single best type of weight-supported exercise for a beginner. Exercise cycles are not very expensive and can be conveniently located in most houses and apartments. From the standpoint of limbic exercise, an exercise cycle offers a beginner an advantage which few other types of exercise do. These exercises allow a person to close his eyes during the exercise with complete safety. *Closing one's eyes* is an absolutely essential element for success in limbic exercise.

A second essential of limbic exercise is the ability to perceive the energy of our body tissues and allow ourselves to be led by it — muscles that contract to produce motion, tendons that convey the tension from muscles to bones, ligaments that hold bones together, and bones that support the muscles. We listen and then respond accordingly. During early training, the tired and listless tissues often tell us to stop. If that happens, we do just that. We listen to them and abide by them. When the legs wish not to move anymore, we do not force them. It may mean that we are not able to exercise for more than a few minutes at a time. An exercise cycle allows us to stop when our legs wish to do so, and begin again, at brief intervals and as many times as we wish. There is no need to dress for it or wear special shoes. There is no need to get to any track. Indeed, there is no need to leave the room. It is especially appropriate for people who suffer from chronic low back pain, neck spasms and stiffness, arthritis, bursitis, myositis and related musculoskeletal disorders.

Swimming is another good weight-supported exercise. Initially, it can help build stamina. It loosens the muscles and frees many of the musculoskeletal restrictions that physically inactive people develop. However, most people cannot fit enough swimming into their schedules, in my view, for optimal health. It is difficult for most people to reap the full benefits of limbic exercise with swimming alone. The central element in limbic exercise I describe in this book is the matter of bringing a spiritual dimension into our mornings. I have tried to emphasize the influence the rising sun and the eastern sky have on the human condition. Swimming as exercise is limited in this regard. Clearly, however, swimming and the eastern sky are not mutually exclusive.

EXPERIMENTATION WITH DIFFERENT EXERCISES

For the beginner, any form of slow and sustained exercise is the right form of exercise — as long as he seeks to perceive the tissues energy and allows himself to be led by it. Wherever the tissues lead us, we let them. The way tissues respond to a particular type of exercise gives us the clues we need. Tissue resistance is equally revealing. Leisure walking, speedwalking, jogging, sprinting, jumping rope, jumping on a trampoline, and exercise with treadmills, steppers and other types of exercise equipment are acceptable forms of exercise for the beginner.

TRY, SENSE AND TRY AGAIN

Those are the key words. Trying, sensing the tissue response and trying again are the necessary elements for success in limbic exercise. The tissues do respond during exercise just as they do during autoregulation performed in a sitting posture. Rotating exercises has the great advantage of inviting many more fibers of connective tissue and muscles to participate. Rotation in exercise, I repeat here, is as necessary in exercise as it is in selection of foods at mealtime.

GUIDANCE FROM WITHIN

The essence of limbic exercise, I indicated earlier, is to seek guidance about exercise from within. While we do not disregard the experience and insights of others, we must be guided by the energy within us. (In the early cortical phase, we listen to others but in the end we listen to ourselves.) It is a good philosophy in other endeavors of life, and it is good philosophy for exercise. Nothing brings this guidance from within more lucidly and with greater force than the limbic energy and limbic images I describe in the chapter Unto the Rising Sun. I know this from my own considerable experience as well as from the true-to-life experiences of my patients who generously shared them with me.

CYCLING TO LIMBIC OPENNESS

For several reasons, I recommend that the beginner start his training for limbic exercise with an exercise cycle. The cycle used should be an inexpensive one without any electronic gimmicks. Flashing, ticking and beeping video screens on exercise equipment are cortical devices, pure and simple. They are completely and utterly irrelevant to our desire to achieve limbic openness through the pursuit of limbic exercise and the language of silence.

Three elements are essential for limbic exercise with an exercise cycle:

First,

we set no goals.

Goals are cortical devices. We do not need them in limbic exercise. In the context of limbic exercise, setting goals for exercise is nothing more than scheming to punish tissues. Consider, for example, the simplest of all goals: duration of exercise. How many of us think of doing exercise for twenty or thirty minutes, look at our watches, and decide that so much time simply cannot be dedicated to exercise that day? How many of us think of how hard we need to drive our muscles, hearts and lungs for the putative cardiovascular and respiratory benefits of exercise? How many of us invest money in expensive futuristic gadgets but seldom, if ever, use such equipment? How many of us see our impulses to do exercise killed by a cortical censor?

Second,

we let our eyes fall upon something and let them stay with it.

The something for the eyes may be a branch of a tree or a twig of a bush visible through a window, a patch of snow or grass, a cloud in the sky, or simply a picture of a flower if no suitable windows are available. With time, the eyes become heavy and want to close.

Third,

we let our eyes close if they wish to do so.

As we learn to keep our cortical monkey out of the way of our eyes, the eyes begin to follow their own inner cues: Sometimes the eyes want to stay closed, and at other times they wish to open. We must simply accept what they choose to do.

I repeat, any exercise is better than no exercise. Thus, exercise done with exercise videos, music or even with TV news has clear physiologic benefits, and will up-regulate fat-burning enzymes. None of these exercises, however, leads us down the path of limbic listening. None of these exercises can banish the cortical monkey. None of these exercises can lead us the way the eastern sky lit by a rising sun does. Exercise with a treadmill clearly is not suitable if our purpose is to seek limbic openness. Treadmills define the pace for the individual and negate the very essence of the limbic state as one that is free of any external programming, restraints or controls.

LIMBIC BURSTS

Sometime during my limbic run I became aware of a physical phenomenon I believe to be universal. I noticed that the speed of my run often changes without any deliberate attempts on my part. My usual limbic run, of course, is a slow, sustained running in place. I make no attempts to achieve any predetermined speed, pulse rate, or any specific breathing rate. Nor is it my purpose to reach any other goals. Yet I notice that at times my legs spontaneously break into a sprint and moments later I recognize this change. Initially, whenever this happened, I'd make deliberate attempts to break this burst and resume my regular pace. After some weeks or months I recognized that even this interference is a device of the cortical monkey in its desperate efforts to regain control over my body. Once I became aware of this interference, I let my limbs lead me. The limbs, I mentioned earlier, do not ever mislead anyone. These bursts of speed interspersed with a slow, sustained run became a natural order of things for me.

Several months later, I read an article written by a professional trainer describing what athletes call interval training. Competitive athletes use this technique to improve their physical endurance. In this technique, they alternate periods of intense physical activity with periods of less intense exercise. The writer of that article detailed many advantages of this particular type of training for athletes. Specifically, he described how interval training in running improves speed as well as stamina. I wondered how athletes might have discovered this phenomenon. Perhaps in the same way I did.

How does interval training — limbic bursts in our lingo — improve speed as well as stamina? The exercise specialist will most likely furnish some elegant mechanical explanations for this. Or, perhaps he will talk about accumulation of fatigue molecules such as lactic acid in muscles as the reason for this phenomenon. Excess lactic acid makes the tissue fluid acidic, and increased acidity impairs the efficiency of energy-generating enzymes. In our autoregulation language, a simple answer, of course, may be that it has something to do with the limbic sense of tissues.

PULSE RATES DURING EXERCISE

Pulse rates during limbic exercise, I indicated earlier, are utterly irrelevant to us. Limbic exercise is about limbic openness. It is about freedom from the demands of the thinking head. It is about opening ourselves to the larger *presence* around us. The pulse table below is included as an example of cleverly crafted tables of the cortical monkey! Pulse counts do nothing but distract us in our reach for the limbic state.

Pulse Table

AGE	70%	85%	MAX
5	150	180	215
10	150	175	210
15	145	170	205
20	140	170	200
25	140	170	200
30	135	165	195
35	132	162	190
40	130	160	185
45	125	155	180
50	115	145	170
55	110	140	165
60	105	135	160
65	105	130	155

All exercise programs carry dangers for the beginner. An excellent method for substantially increasing this danger is to push ourselves in exercise to reach a predetermined pulse rate.

*"My trainer insists I count, but when I count
my blood pressure goes up."*

A schoolteacher who suffers from high blood pressure
spoke these words during a visit with me.

"So what do you do?" I asked.
"I count when he looks at me," he replied.
"And when he is not looking at you?"
"I close my eyes and quit counting."
"Why?"
"Because I like it better that way."

This is a problem I often encounter. People want to
follow their own impulses. The experts do not let them.

CALORIC EXPENDITURE WITH ACTIVITIES

The table on the next page gives the number of calories
used per hour for metabolic activities.

Activities	Calories
Sleeping	80
Sitting	100
Driving	120
Standing	140
Household work	180
Walking 2.5 mph*	210
Walking 4 mph	360
Walking 5 mph	585
Gardening	220
Swimming	300
Running	900

* Walking at two and half MPH requires 210 calories per hour

To burn off 1 pound of fat, a person needs to utilize about 4,000 calories — that means he will need to walk about 19 miles.

Interestingly, this table explains why people who seek to lose weight by exercise alone never succeed on a long-term basis. For example, a person would need to run for two hours to burn the calories contained in a meal consisting of a cheeseburger, French fries and apple pie. After running two hours, he will be tired and hungry enough to want to eat a similar meal all over again.

I repeat, limbic exercise is not about burning off calories. It is done to up-regulate fat-burning enzymes — lipases and other enzymes. This is a critically important issue and I repeat it several times in this volume. Up-regulated fat-burning enzymes burn fat efficiently even when the individual is sleeping. By contrast, down-regulated fat-burning enzymes allow build up of fat even when the individual is exercising. Loss of excess weight and achievement of life span weight follows as a natural course of events when we keep our fat-burning enzymes up-regulated with life span food choices and with limbic exercise.

RUG RUNNING

Earlier in this chapter I describe how I do my limbic run every morning for 15 to 30 minutes. I run in place. A small three foot by three foot area rug keeps me anchored to the small area where I wish to stay.

I wake up in the morning and begin my day with a deep sense of gratitude for being alive and being able to spring out of bed with palpable energy. As I wrote earlier, I consider being able to get out of bed a cause for celebration. I know many people who are unable to perform this simple task. Just out of bed, and on some occasions while in it, I rub the tissues in my neck and shoulders and spend one or two minutes doing reverse isometric exercises for my neck muscles as outlined in the chapter The Rooster and Limbic Lengthening. After this I take my daily supplements. *Everyone must.* As long as we breathe in polluted air all day long and take a bolus of contaminants with each meal, nutrients are essential to provide a counterbalance.

This viewpoint is supported by all serious students of human biology. Physicians who practice drug medicine and consider nutritional medicine quackery are pathetically uninformed about the real issues of nutrition we face today. I discuss this subject at length in *The Butterfly and Life Span Nutrition.*

I usually take about 16 ounces of water with my supplements. Five days a week, my breakfast consists of one and a half heaping tablespoons of a peptide and protein formulation mixed with vegetable juices. Uncommonly, I mix this formula with fruit juices. This gives me another 16 ounces of fluid before I step out on a covered patio for my daily limbic run. The patio offers protection from rain, snow or very cold air in winter. I do not make any preparations for exercise. I do not need any special exercise attire.

I begin jogging in place, slowly taking the lead from my limbs. Within several moments, I find myself leaning against the brick wall of the patio, doing limbic lengthening steps for my upper and lower back, shoulders and thigh muscles as outlined in the preceding chapter. I do not consciously follow any techniques nor do I set any time limits. Some minutes pass, and I find myself back into running in place on my rug. My eyes usually settle on some object — a twig, a berry on a bush, a patch of snow, a bird on a ledge, or a patch of grass. Sooner or later, my eyes reach for some clouds in the eastern sky. Sometimes they peer into the deep clearing above the low-lying clouds. Some more moments pass and my eyes want to close. Sometimes my movements change into those of jumping rope. It is as if someone drops a rope. (No rope really appears. My limbs make their own decision. Years ago I started out with a rope but I kept misplacing the rope. Then my limbs freed me from the need for a rope — they go through the motion of jumping with a rope very well without requiring a rope.) Then follow some limbic bursts. My limbs move with different speeds and change the patterns of motion from a slow ghoraa run to little sprints and settle back into a ghoraa run again. My legs, loin and lower abdominal muscles find their own rhythm. My eyes close and open and close again, following some unknown leads.

I used to take a watch out with me. It gave me some measure of time. Now I do not. My limbs do not need it. The cortical monkey still asks for it sometimes. Morning is not a time for my monkey — and my monkey knows that (I think). After the run I come back into the house for some upper body muscle-building exercises. I do some work with weights or do some push-ups, again taking the lead of my limbs.

THE CORTICAL MONKEY CRAVES CLOCKS

The cortical monkey adores watches. It loves to watch the second and minute arms on the dial. The limbic impulses of our roosters know how to deal with the infatuation of our monkeys with watches. A beginner, however, may have to learn to confront the cortical monkey with some cortical devices — give him a taste of his own medicine. I repeat, we do not set any goals, no goals for time, no goals for speed, no goals for technique. We do not fall for the trick of planning exercise for 20 minutes, or 15 minutes or 10 minutes. Simply let the limbic limbs lead you. If it can be only two minutes, let it be. Four minutes? Let it be. I know from long personal experience — as well as the experience of many of my patients — that limbic impulses do drown out the cortical screams when we learn to let them.

PUSH-UPS AND SIT-UPS

It is useful to add some push-ups and sit-ups to our daily limbic exercise. These types of exercise clearly are glycolytic or sugar-burning in nature and do not help us much in up-regulation of fat-burning exercise. However, both exercises offer the advantage of putting into motion a very large number of muscles, ligaments and tendons. These exercises are useful for freeing many musculoskeletal restrictions that commonly develop during the sleeping hours. To avoid sudden stresses on unwarmed and unprepared tissues, it is advisable to do these exercises at the end of the regular limbic exercise.

Push-ups are an excellent exercise. No equipment is required. Any place is the right place. Any length of time is the right duration for this exercise. If the general condition of the individual allows, push-ups should be a part of his morning. If push-ups seem too strenuous, one can use appropriate weights. Above all, exercise must be *slow* and *sustained.*

Sit-ups are excellent exercises for the abdominal and leg muscles just as push-ups are for the arm muscles. As I write this my thoughts return to Kirto, my village in Pakistan. There were some superb athletes among the boys then. All the equipment they ever needed were the fields. Running, sit-ups and push-ups were all the scientific exercises they ever did. Mother Earth! Winds from the distant lands! A rising sun! Those were the elements. The boys had it all. No one ever told them they needed special shoes. No one cautioned them against running without spandex. Their complete attire was a loin cloth deftly wrapped around their waists. There were no graphs, no pie charts, no score cards, and certainly none of this nonsense about 70% percentile of Max_2. It amuses me to realize that after some decades of extensive study of the technology of Stars Wars medicine, I have turned to the three things I know best: simple running, sit-ups and push-ups.

I do my push-ups and sit-ups after the limbic run when my body tissues are warmed up and energized for more demanding work. Strenuous exercises like push-ups should be undertaken only when the state of musculoskeletal conditioning allows them with safety.

DIRECTED PULSES

Directed pulses are the ability to bring about selective vasodilatation (opening up of the arteries to increase blood and energy flow) in different parts of the body. For most people, hands are the first parts of the body to respond to self-regulatory methods. This is the reason why hand warming has been one of the basic techniques used throughout history. In my clinical work, the perception of pulsations in fingertips can be verified as a physiologic change (vasodilation) with an instrument called a plethysmograph. Directed pulses then is the learned ability to cause the blood vessels in a desired part of the body to dilate.

The method of directed pulses is simple and extremely useful for training in autoregulation. I discuss the methods and the effects of directed pulses in *The Limbic Dog and Directed Pulses.* To do directed pulses during limbic exercise, one must first learn to do directed pulses at rest. For this, I suggest the reader consult *The Limbic Dog and Directed Pulses* and consider training in autoregulation with a knowledgeable and experienced professional. Alternatively, he may wish to use the tape I prepared for my own patients (available from the Institute).

The simple sequence of sentences used in the initial training of directed pulses and other methods of autoregulation can be used as effortlessly during the exercise as during regular autoregulation done in a sitting position. With little effort, the verbal cues sink in with the natural rhythm of the leg, loin and shoulder muscles. The tissues respond to limbic listening with varying expressions of energy during exercise just as they do with self-regulation in a sitting position.

LIMBIC BREATHING FOR LIMBIC EXERCISE

In *The Cortical Monkey and Healing,* I described limbic

breathing as a specific type of breathing that is of enormous value for autoregulation and healing. I, and many of my patients, have also found this type of breathing of great value in limbic exercise. I refer the reader to the chapter Lata and Limbic Breathing in that book for a detailed description of limbic breathing. Here I include some brief comments about it and illustrate its essential element.

In limbic breathing, each breath is taken to achieve a well-defined objective. In early training, a person uses limbic breathing to become aware of the process of breathing. Next, limbic breathing is practiced to dissolve the feelings of anxiety and anger and to control the stress response. With more training, limbic breathing is used to learn control over the functions of the heart, arteries, brain, skin and other organs. With still more extensive experience, this mode of breathing is the most effective method for the initial work of self-healing. Finally, limbic breathing ushers a person into higher states of consciousness.

Limbic breathing has three essential aspects: 1) a slow, sustained breathe-out; 2) diaphragmatic breathing; and 3) perception of energy in body tissues during the prolonged breathe-out period. In the following diagram, I illustrate the relationship between the breathe-in, brief hold and breathe-out phases of limbic breathing.

Cortical Breathing

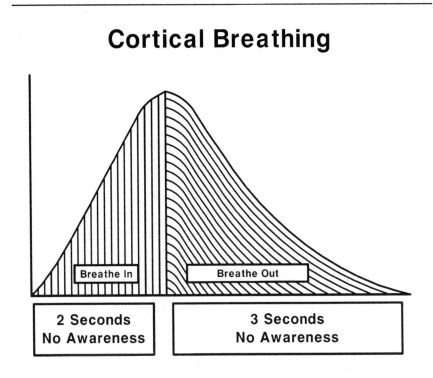

Breathe In

Breathe Out

| 2 Seconds No Awareness | 3 Seconds No Awareness |

Limbic Breathing
Advanced

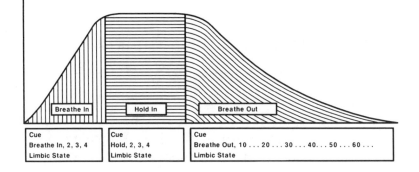

Breathe In

Hold In

Breathe Out

| Cue Breathe In, 2, 3, 4 Limbic State | Cue Hold, 2, 3, 4 Limbic State | Cue Breathe Out, 10 . . . 20 . . . 30 . . . 40 . . . 50 . . . 60 . . . Limbic State |

The emphasis on the role and efficacy of breathing in the various methods for autoregulation is not new. The central role of various breathing methods in the meditative techniques of Egyptian priests, Hindu yogis, Buddhist teachers, Tibetan lamas, Christian monks and Muslim sufies and dervishes are well documented.

The language of biology is energy. The language of molecules is oxidation and reduction. Oxygen breaks molecules down to smaller sizes and releases energy for various life processes; reduction builds them back and stores energy. Oxidation, by and large, requires oxygen. We breathe oxygen to sustain life. For the professional reader, I have discussed the essentials of the chemistry and energy generation at the cell membrane in my monograph *The Agony and Death of a Cell* published in the 1991 syllabus of the American Academy of Environmental Medicine.

What is often not fully understood is that the modes of breathing (and changes in the pattern of oxygen utilization brought about by them) profoundly influence the energy, molecular and cellular functions in our tissues.

THINKING ABOUT HOW NOT TO THINK: A CATCH 22

For limbic openness, we must first be freed from the relentless censor of the cortical monkey. Switching off the thinking cortical mode is simple to understand at an intellectual level, but it requires considerable practical skill in real life situations. This is a universal experience. Limbic breathing, when mastered and practiced frequently, is the simplest and most effective method for shutting out the unrelenting clutter of the cortical mode.

The entry into the limbic mode requires that we ablate all *cortical thoughts.* This is easier said than done. It is a classic catch 22 situation: thinking about how not to think. It is a competitive effort. The harder one tries not to think, the deeper into thinking he slides. All competitive functions are cortical functions; trying hard not to think assures continuity in thinking.

Limbic breathing, once learned well, is very useful in the early stages of limbic exercise.

THE ROOSTER DIES —
THE CORTICAL MONKEY LIVES

I return to the rooster. I wonder what goals the rooster sets when he flaps his wings to announce the morning? How does he pace his wing flapping? How does he determine when to speed up and when to slow down? How does he know when to stop? The rooster has a message for us: His wings *know* and so do our limbs.

How many of us wish we could exercise each morning?

How many of us feel such a natural, spontaneous and limbic urge? Before we can allow the limbs to lead, the cortical monkey intervenes. We look at the watch and begin to talk to ourselves. "Twenty minutes? No! I don't have that kind of time. Maybe fifteen minutes? No! Not really! Ten minutes? Hardly! Just five minutes? Don't be silly! What would monkeying around for five minutes really do? Don't you remember reading about that medical study. That *definitively* proves that to gain any benefits from exercise, you have to exercise for at least twenty minutes. I mean, that's when endorphins are really released. What good is exercise if you cannot feel the endorphin high? High! That's it. I mean a *high* is what I really need right now, don't I? Yes! That' it. Something to pick me up. Something to give me a high. And it can't be exercise. Not today, in any case. Coffee! Yes! That's it! Today it must be coffee. Black coffee. Hot black coffee. That's it. That is what I really need today. Tomorrow will be a different day. Tomorrow it may be exercise. Maybe I'll even try Ali's limbic thing."

The rooster dies. The cortical monkey lives.

ENERGY-OVER-MIND STILLNESS

Autoregulation, I indicated earlier in this volume, is not about the popular — and in my view erroneous — mind-over-body concept of health and disease. Autoregulation is about the energy of living tissues. It is about visceral calm, an energetic stillness. It is about the absence of relentless thinking. It is about an "energy-over-mind" stillness.

Canceling cortical clutter is the essence of limbic exercise. For the trainee, I recommend two methods that I have observed to be most effective during my work with autoregulation: the method of directed pulses and the method of limbic breathing.

****

In closing this chapter, let me emphasize the critical difference between cortical greed and limbic gratitude. Limbic exercise is not about a struggle for some "70 percentile pulse" or for some target breathing rate, or for scores that our exercise experts ask us to keep. All this is cortical greed, simple and pure. Limbic exercise is about openness and about limbic gratitude. It is about a spiritual dimension in our lives.

"Out of pain grow the violets of patience and sweetness. The richness of the human experience would lose something of rewarding joy if there were no limitations to overcome."

Helen Keller

Chapter 9

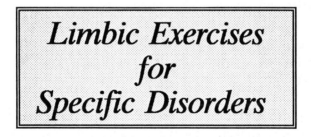

Limbic Exercises
for
Specific Disorders

The limbic state is an energy state. It can exist only when the cortical monkey has been banished. The principle of autoregulation requires that we learn to become aware of tissue energy, perceive how this energy is amplified and become sensitive to how it directs itself to different tissues. Autoregulation requires that we acquire a sensitivity to the tissues in duress. This principal is as pertinent to limbic exercise as it is to autoregulation done for other healing phenomena.

Different body organs serve as "spokesorgans" for different individuals. Sometimes, it seems that the spokesorgan is elected by other organs, at other times it appears more likely that the genes sensing the trouble select an organ to convey the body's message. When the spokesorgan hurts, it often expresses the pain of many other organs. A state of disease, with rare exceptions, is not an abrupt departure from a state of health. A state of absence of health evolves slowly from a state of health. Chronic diseases, as they are known today, are tail-end events — in essence, the consequences of the impact of environmental factors on the genetic makeup. Looking at body organs under duress as spokesorgans fundamentally changes the way we look at illnesses.

In autoregulation, the issues of technique, training, time and perfection of skills become irrelevant once we learn to perceive the energy of life and allow it to lead us. However, in my work with autoregulation training sessions for my patients and students, I have observed that some methods of training yield clearly superior initial results than others. The choice of the method, time and setting of training profoundly influences the outcome. The same considerations hold when we seek to do autoregulation concurrently with physical exercise. This is the *first essential consideration* in limbic exercise for the beginner.

Different tissues are injured in different ways. Injured tissues respond differently to different insults. Evidently, the needs of a hurt heart are quite different from those of the bones thinned out by osteoporosis. In this sense, the fitness needs of a joint damaged by arthritis are distinct from those of muscles weakened by disuse atrophy. These are important considerations for individuals who suffer from various health disorders as they begin limbic exercise. This is the *second essential consideration* in limbic exercise for those who suffer from chronic disorders. However, all this becomes irrelevant when he succeeds in allowing his limbic impulses to guide him along. A third consideration is the matter of recognizing and interpreting signals from the injured tissues — the spokesorgan of the body.

SIGNALS FROM SPOKESORGANS

The essence of limbic exercise is absence of focus and perception of energy. In chronic illness, it is necessary for the beginner to heed the signals from the spokesorgan of the body. Some methods of self-regulation are more effective than others in preventing additional stress on the body organs suffering from chronic illness. To this end, I make some suggestions concerning the types of autoregulation methods that add safety to exercise in specific chronic disorders and improve the benefits that are expected from limbic exercise. This is especially pertinent for the beginner. With time, the limbic mode takes over and there is no need to make conscious efforts to use one or the other method of self-regulation while doing limbic exercise. Energy flows spontaneously and freely. I discuss my recommendations for specific limbic exercise for various health disorders in the following order:

1. Heart disease
2. Hypertension
3. Anxiety state and panic attacks
4. Depression
5. Arthritis, bursitis and related disorders
6. Osteoporosis
7. Gastrointestinal disorders
8. Disorders of the troubled trio
      The injured thyroid
      The overburdened pancreas
      The chronically stressed adrenal
9. Asthma and respiratory disorders
10. Chronic fatigue
11. Old age
12. Obesity

Before I make some specific suggestions about each of the above disorders, I want to make some brief comments about the central issues in exercise today: fatigue, stress, anxiety, anger, inertia, stiff and unyielding connective tissue, limp muscles, sore tissues, injured organs, and a dispirited view of life. These are the real impediments to exercise. These are the elements that give teeth to the bites of the limbic dog. Pursuit of physical fitness for a longer, healthier life with exercise simply seems too onerous.

LIVING WITH THE LIMBIC DOG

Just as limbic pacing is the key to success in limbic exercise for the healthy, coping with the bites of the limbic dog is the stumbling block in limbic exercise for the chronically ill. Limbic openness with limbic exercise comes effortlessly and naturally to some yet eludes others.

Some of my patients who take my workshop for limbic exercise try a ghoraa run on a piece of rug or ride an exercise cycle with closed eyes. They return and describe their discovery of the exhilaration of motion for motion's sake — different senses of movement, new perceptions of space, changing relationships with the world around them. They speak of primal experiences — recall with some shape and texture the elements of early man's discoveries. They sense what he felt when he looked to the sky to search for the meaning of his existence and when he closed his eyes to reach within for what he couldn't see with open eyes. They describe how slow, sustained motion with no focus transports them to a state of deep, visceral calm — a stillness that transcends the physical and mostly difficult world that surrounds them. They describe images they see, and how those images alter states of consciousness. The discovery that this native-visceral state brings forth new and changing perceptions of life and spirituality is, of course, neither new nor confined to any specific state of consciousness. These are images of man and his relationship to the larger world he lives in — his links with his ghosts and his spirits and the greater *presence* that he cannot see but knows exists all around him.

WHEN WE KNOW SOMETHING, WE CANNOT UNKNOW IT

In limbic exercise, what begins as exercise for fitness or for losing weight is transformed into ever-changing images of light, life and love. Once we *know* such dimensions exist, we cannot "unknow" them. The path, in and of itself, becomes the guiding light. Some other people are not so fortunate. Their search for limbic openness only brings them the anguish of failure; persistence in such search seems to bring only persistent suffering. With each misstep, the bites of the limbic dog become more frequent and sharper. *With patience and time, however, everyone does succeed in reaching the limbic state.* In the chapter The Cortical Monkey and the Limbic Dog, I relate true-to-life case histories of Edward and Sheila, two patients who endured their suffering for long periods before the bites of the limbic dog ceased and their tissues began to respond to them.

LIMBIC EXERCISE FOR HEART DISEASE

For heart disease, I recommend using directed pulses,

ghoraa run and limbic cycling.

There is no better way to gain an awareness of heart function than by perceiving the heartbeat limbically. Heart disease is the number one killer in the United States. Bad advice about physical fitness to people who suffer from heart disease is also the number one folly practiced in cardiac rehabilitation centers nationwide.

> *"Dr. Ali, my husband won't have it any other way. He absolutely insists I follow the pulse number on my treadmill. I really want to close my eyes and do it your way. But he is adamant. He pushes me and pushes me until I reach the number he wants. He had a heart attack recently. He is very rigid about the way his cardiologist wants it. And he is very rigid about it with me. I don't want to stress him anymore. So I give in."*

JK, a woman in her sixties, spoke the above words during a visit. She had obtained little if any benefit from coronary angioplasty, had been advised to have coronary bypass surgery, but instead chose to receive chelation treatment from me.

The cortical monkey prevails everywhere. How many people who suffer from heart disease are being relentlessly driven by their trainers? How many people must have lost their lives in pursuit of the silly numerical goals set up by those in the fitness business? I wonder.

A PHYSICIAN DIES ON A SIDEWALK

Some years ago, one of my physician-friends in his mid-fifties saw his physician for a routine physical. His blood cholesterol level turned out to be moderately high. He was told that an elevated cholesterol level was a significant risk factor for heart disease. He smoked, and that, he was warned, added to the risk of heart attack. His physician prescribed a cholesterol-lowering drug and advised him to reduce the stress in his life. We physicians are very fond of prescribing relaxation. We seldom ask ourselves the key question: If the patient knew how to relax, why wouldn't he? *The essential issue is not that people do not realize they need to relax, it is that they do not know how to relax.*

On his return from his physician's office, my physician-friend was all revved up about lowering his blood cholesterol by running. He chose sidewalk running. Within some days of beginning his running program, he developed a cardiac arrhythmia and collapsed on the street, barely a few hundred yards from the hospital. By the time paramedics reached him, he was dead, a victim of a misguided and fatal assault on a phantom cholesterol problem.

We physicians generally look at heart disease as a plumbing problem — zap it with lasers, blast it with radio waves, roto-rooter it, and if all that doesn't work, bypass it. Then come our fancy exercise machines, fitted with all the bells and whistles and flashes and burps of Star Wars technology — arm ergometers, bicycle ergometers, treadmills and all. The warriors of Star Wars medicine will not have it any other way. They talk about "six-level protocol for monitored phase II cardiac rehabilitation."

Complication rates were initially described as lower in exercise programs with continuous ECG monitoring ...... to ensure that it (heart rate) remains in the prescribed range and to concomitantly estimate their exercise intensity; this may be documented by use of the defibrillator paddles as ECG leads.

The Heart, Page 1111, parenthesis added
McGraw-Hill, New York, 1990.

This is an illuminating bit of text from a leading American textbook of cardiology. Do these heart experts know how people feel when they are wired and made to perform? Examined and scrutinized as if they were experimental animals in research laboratories? Do they ever think what the sight of defibrillator paddles might do to someone who suffers from heart disease? The whole body convulses when those defibrillator paddles are used. Do they think their patients do not know that?

How does exercise of moderate to severe intensity affect the heart? It is generally not realized that moderate and intense exercise increases the activity of the sympathetic nervous system, speeds up the heart rate and raises blood pressure. The degree of sympathetic stimulation — the same response as is seen in physical and emotional stress — is roughly proportional to the intensity of exercise, and blood pressure often increases 40 to 60 mm Hg. Add to this the trauma of being wired up and the horror of seeing defibrillator paddles, and you have a prisoner of Star Wars medicine. We physicians are too wrapped up in our technology gimmicks to see the absurdity in all this.

A heart knows what it wants to do if only we let it. First and foremost, it yearns for freedom, freedom from ECG electrodes, freedom from defibrillator paddles and freedom from the frivolous notions of our cardiac rehabilitation experts. A heart wants to follow its own natural cadence, its own innate rhythm. It wants liberty, a choice to extend itself as much as it sees fit or not at all. The safest exercise for patients with heart disease is limbic exercise with limbic breathing.

LIMBIC BREATHING
GIVES THE ESSENTIAL SAFETY MARGIN

Limbic breathing, by its very nature, will not allow the heart to come under any real stress. The slower the rate of limbic breathing, the greater the safety margin. The inverse also applies: the greater the difficulty in doing limbic breathing, the higher the risk to the heart. Limbic breathing reduces the oxidant stress on the heart at a cellular, energetic level, and does not allow a person to exceed the safe limits of the heart. It is the surest way to abrogate the cortical overdrive that is almost always present (though not often recognized) in our goal-oriented exercise programs.

The common advice of pushing the pulse rate to the 70th percentile of the maximum rate during exercise, it seems to me, is just the wrong advice for people afflicted by heart disease. It completely ignores the margin of safety for the *individual* with heart disease. Indeed, the 70th percentile may prove fatal for some and insufficient for others. In fact, the whole idea of a fixed numerical value for the heart rate that should be achieved during exercise is both frivolous and dangerous — it is destined to take a person to the only place where he or she shouldn't be: a cortical, calculating, competing and stressful state.

LIMBIC EXERCISE FOR HYPERTENSION

For hypertension, I recommend ghoraa run or limbic cycling with methods of limbic dimension.

Limbic dimensions transcend the restrictions imposed on us by the cortical mind. I describe the methods of limbic dimension in *The Limbic Dog and Directed Pulses*. A beginner needs to become proficient in basic methods of autoregulation such as directed pulses and limbic breathing before attempting

these more advanced methods. Still, I suggest the following
simple steps:

1. Sit comfortably and upright in a chair with eyes closed.
2. Softly repeat the words, "I can imagine the space in the back of my
   throat," five times.
3. "Feel" the space in the back of your throat as you gently breathe in
   and out five times.
4. Perceive how the space in the back of your throat responds as you
   breathe in and out.
5. Softly repeat the words, "I feel the space in the back of my
   throat open up as I breathe in and come back together as
   I breathe out," five times.
6. Alternate step # 2 and # 4 for a few moments until the throat
   begins to respond as you breathe in and out.

The above exercise may be done by perceiving the
energy of other tissues and with the spaces in and between
other organs such as eyes or ears or other body organs. Most of
my patients perceive changing dimensions with these methods
the first time they follow the above steps with me in my
autoregulation laboratory. The purpose of such exercises is to
break through the limitations we impose upon our senses.
Initially, changing limbic dimensions clearly carry the illusion of
changes in the dimension of space behind the throat or between
other body organs. In time, we move from simple illusions to
perceptions of real tissue energy.

Hypertension, high blood pressure in common language,
is a silent killer that has virtually no symptoms in its early stages
and often remains unrecognized for years. The individual with
hypertension suffers no pain and sees no need for medical care.
Sadly, the problem during early years is often made worse by us

physicians who make the diagnosis and use this diagnostic label as a license to dole out drugs.

Hypertension is nothing but tightened arteries. The arteries tighten when they are intimidated; they literally *shrink* away from the threat. Arteries in hypertension are often recalcitrant. Early borderline hypertension generally responds well to self-regulation, appropriate changes in nutrition and slow, sustained exercise. This, however, does not hold for people with established hypertension of moderate to severe degree. Such individuals have to be patient, and be prepared to face the bites of the limbic dog. On a positive note, almost all people can reduce the amounts of drugs they use for control of hypertension with autoregulation. On occasion, I have even observed normalization of raised blood pressure with persistent use of nutrients and self-regulation in severe cases. Hypertension caused by rare tumors and advanced autoimmune disorders, of course, is a different problem.

"Drugs do not seem to help, gym does make a difference. Going to gym does it — it drops my blood pressure 30 to 40 points."

The above words were spoken by a school teacher whose blood pressure ranged from 150/90 to 220/115. His physician had tried a host of antihypertensive drugs with poor results. Within several weeks of starting nutrient therapies, autoregulation and limbic exercise, he told me his blood pressure in most days was well below the upper limit of normality of 140/90.

LIMBIC EXERCISE FOR ANXIETY
STATES AND PANIC ATTACKS

For these disorders, I recommend aerobic exercises done with suitable videos and in classes organized by local spas in the early stages. After the initial period, ghoraa run and limbic cycling, in my view, are the best exercises.

Anxiety states and panic attacks are common disorders caused by molecular roller coasters. Adrenergic hypervigilence — unnecessary and unrestricted productions of adrenaline and related stress molecules — is the earmark of our time. The common stress state — that everyone recognizes so readily and experts find so hard to define — is not simply a matter of too many adrenaline molecules. It is a *state* of molecular feeding frenzy — the chemistry of the fireworks of the fourth of July that includes cholinergic surges, sharp peaks and deep lows of neurotransmitters, bursts of insulin and sparks of electro-magnetic energy. For acute distress, drugs are very effective for control of symptoms. Over the long haul, however, drugs give poor results. For chronic symptoms, nutritional therapies, effective methods of self-regulation and limbic exercise offer the best results. No one, in my view, can hope to obtain lasting relief from these disorders without limbic breathing and doing slow, sustained exercise as the centerpiece for his strategy.

The simple act of closing one's eyes is stressful for many people who suffer chronic anxiety and panic attacks. This is the main reason I recommend that such individuals begin their exercise with some external support provided by suitable exercise videos or in classes organized in their local spas. As the symptoms abate, such individuals begin to discover the deeply restorative calm that can only come with closed eyes and a limbic, visceral stillness.

LIMBIC EXERCISE FOR DEPRESSION

For depression, my recommendation is similar to that for anxiety state: aerobic exercise with suitable videos or in classes at local spas during the early stages and ghoraa run with limbic breathing later on.

For crisis management in life-threatening suicidal depression, drugs and electroconvulsive therapy are generally necessary. Deep depression is generally a very difficult problem to manage without drugs. However, this can be achieved in most cases. As in the case of anxiety states and panic attacks, long-term success requires an integrated strategy that includes nutritional therapies, effective methods of self-regulation, environmental therapies and limbic exercise.

For best long-term results, however, no therapy is as effective as limbic breathing and limbic exercise. This may seem like strange advice to some patients as well as professionals, but this is what I have learned from my patients who suffered from severe depression that proved refractory to all standard drug therapies.

I include the case history of Edward and the story of the gray dog in the chapter The Cortical Monkey and Limbic Dog in this book for a specific purpose. People in the throes of insufferable suffering should know their tissues may not warm up to them on short order. Creating hope for them is usually easy, sustaining it until energy responses emerge often proves difficult. The suffering of those who suffer from severe depression has no limits. It robs them of the very will and endurance they need to fight back with. In the section on the Fields of Candles in the above-mentioned chapter, I draw an analogy to illustrate the essential neurochemical abnormalities that cause depression. The bites of the limbic dog are often sharp and insufferable in severe depression.

The simple act of closing the eyes deepens the darkness that is the agony of depression. Such agony requires some special considerations. For the victims of persistent depression, participation in group exercises often becomes necessary. A lesser choice is the use of exercise videos.

Almost all of my patients who suffer from severe depression eventually reach a stage when they can close their eyes without deepening their depression. Limbic exercise, then, becomes superior to all other types of exercise. The language of silence allows an escape from their silos of sadness.

In depression, the morning hours are usually difficult. It is a time when they lack most what they need most: the capacity to break through the hold of dark, restless night hours. Nothing will pull them out of the paralyzing darkness of depression more than the gentle guiding energy of a rising sun. There can be no substitute for the eastern sky on clear days for them. Improbable as it may seem, the best medicine for securing deep sleep for people who suffer depression is limbic exercise done the morning before.

LIMBIC EXERCISE FOR ARTHRITIS

For arthritis, myositis, chronic myofascial trigger points and related disorders, I recommend limbic cycling.

The principle of limbic exercise for people who suffer from arthritis and related disorders is the same as for those who do not. However, there are some differences in applications. Individuals with arthritis require a longer period of slow but sustained warm-up. Adequate limbic lengthening and stretching of muscles, ligaments and tendons significantly reduce the risk of tearing the fibers in these tissues. There is some evidence that the water content of the cartilage lining the joints increases during early periods of exercise, reducing the potential of further injury to the underlying bone. The intensity and duration of exercise and whether exercise is weight-supported or weight-bearing exercises are other important issues for people who suffer from such disorders. Swimming and exercise programs in heated water (temperature between 78-82°F) are of great value for such patients. Other exercises chosen must also be of the no- or low-impact type.

Some exercise experts assert that the "ideal" minimum walking pace should be "as low as 40 percent of maximum oxygen consumption." Such *numerical shackles* are of no relevance to our discussion of limbic exercise. The core idea of limbic exercise is this: We perceive *the* tissue energy. The tissues *know* how fast or how far or how long they wish to move. All we have to do is let them lead the way. Sometimes the tissues wish to move briskly. If they do, so be it. If they wish to move more leisurely, that's okay too.

Forty percent of oxygen consumption, to be candid, is foolish advice for the arthritis sufferer. For one thing, how does a person in the throes of chronic joint and connective tissue disorders know what constitutes 100% of his maximal oxygen consumption? If he doesn't know what 100% is, how can he compute 40%?

Elastic support for tender tissues during limbic exercise is an excellent idea. These supports keep the tissues warm and protect them from injury by restricting the range of motion of involved joints. Some rheumatologist recommend the use of nonsteroidal anti-inflammatory drugs (NSAIDs) for exercise, even when the person with arthritis doesn't take drugs routinely (*New Jersey Medicine* 88:657; 1991). This is precisely opposite to what limbic exercise is all about. Dulling the pain with drugs for exercise? Eliminating the protective pain mechanisms so that yet more injury can be inflicted on the damaged joint tissues? That's one clear example of how our drug thinking clouds our judgment. It is strange advice coming from a rheumatologist who should know better.

LIMBIC EXERCISE FOR OSTEOPOROSIS

For prevention and reversal of osteoporosis, I recommend jumping on a trampoline or jumping rope.

Our milk industry has done a fantastic job of convincing all of us that osteoporosis is a calcium disorder that is best cured by drinking copious quantities of milk or eating thick chunks of cheese. Makers of calcium pills were inspired by the financial success of the milk industry. They hopped on the bandwagon of calcium. We physicians know calcium does not work for osteoporosis. We simply go along because nutrition, for the most part, is of no interest to us.

Osteoporosis is loss of bone matter. Minerals in bones are poorly deposited. The bone spicules become thin. Weakened bones bend to produce increased back curvatures and in extreme forms, hunchbacks. Finally, such bones break with minimal trauma.

There is something amusing about the opinions of medical experts on the payroll of the dairy industry. When I do autopsies on old women who die of various causes, I almost always see heavy deposits of calcium in their arteries and moderate to severe osteoporosis. Evidently, calcium exists in abundance where it is not needed and is deficient where it is. Calcium overload in arteries suffocates tissues at the same time that insufficient calcium — and some other minerals — deposits in bones leads to osteoporosis, bone deformity and fractures. Osteoporosis experts who write tomes about bone weakness never write about this paradox.

The commonly held view is that osteoporosis results from inadequate supply of the female hormone, estrogen. I have serious reservations about this simplistic view. A *functional "hyperestrogenic" state* is one of the major issues for women today. It is progesterone — the hormone that provides counterbalance to estrogen — that should be of concern to us. I discuss this subject at length in my forthcoming book, *What Do Woodpeckers Know About Osteoporosis?* Here I make the essential point about the true cause of osteoporosis in one simple sentence: Osteoporosis is caused by oxidative damage to the hormone receptors and other molecules in bone that are intricately involved in the deposition of calcium, phosphorus, magnesium, boron and other minerals as well as in the laying down of the protein matrix of bone. Milk and cheese as sources of calcium can be consumed until the cows come home, but it will not cure osteoporosis. It is that simple!

If oxidative molecular injury to bone is the cause of osteoporosis, what are the rational strategies for its reversal? There are three essentials here: 1) slow, sustained exercise that puts direct healthy stress on the axial skeleton (vertebrae in the neck, upper back and lower back) and promotes bone remodeling and new bone formation; 2) normalization of hormonal imbalance with natural progesterone therapy; and 3) life span foods that provide counterbalance to aging-oxidant molecules in our internal and external environment. I devote *The Butterfly and Life Span Nutrition* to the subject of life span foods. Here I make some comments regarding some specific aspects of exercise that are essential for reversing osteoporosis.

> *Until more evidence is in, it probably would be unwise to recommend aerobic exercise solely to prevent osteoporosis.*

Postgraduate Medicine 90:106; 1991

When I first read the above lines, I did a double-take. I read it again and then a third time. *It probably would be unwise to recommend aerobic exercise!* Medical students are generally intelligent people. I know because I went to school with them. What is it about our medical education system that depletes us of common sense? I often wonder. We enter medical schools as rational, inquisitive students of human biology; we emerge as practitioners who begin with the name of a disease and end with the name of a drug. Is there another man, woman or child alive in the world — other than a physician — who would make a silly statement like the one quoted above? Why would the author of this article, a physician who heads a department of family medicine in a Midwestern hospital, make an absurd statement like this? The probable answer is that he is trying to be what he believes is a good *medical scientist.* Since he cannot come up with a suitable double-blind cross-over study to show the right numbers, he has chosen to be scientifically pure and pristine. Scientifically, pure and pristine and *dead,* as Sinclair Lewis would have put it.

In reality, regular exercise increases bone density in women at all ages from 20 to 80 (Bone Miner 1:115; 1986), and exercise, physical fitness, and muscle strength all correlate with bone density in premenopausal and postmenopausal women and in men aged 30 to 75 (reviewed in BMJ 303:453; 1991). There are many more studies that can be cited to document the good effects of exercise on osteoporosis. The key to success is a special program of exercise that promotes new bone formation.

Bone is a living tissue. Ongoing bone resorption, new bone formation and modelling are integral to life. Physical activity decreases bone resorption and promotes new bone formation. The critical element in this context is that the newly formed bone models itself in response to need — the nature and intensity of the strain and stress on the bone defines the demand for strength and determines how the bone spicules are aligned and re-aligned for strength and resilience.

For the prevention and reversal of osteoporosis, we need to put direct, low-grade, repetitive stress along the axis of alignment. In other words, we need to put remodeling stress on the bone in the direction we want to build strength. Thus, for strengthening the vertebral and thigh bones — the frequent sites of fractures — the ideal exercises are jumping with a rope or on a trampoline.

LIMBIC EXERCISE FOR GASTROINTESTINAL DISORDERS AND BLOATING

For chronic problems of the bowel and for excessive

flatulence and bloating, I recommend methods of limbic dimension, ghoraa run and jumping rope in the morning.

There are three important issues here: 1) how to prevent excessive gas formation in the bowel; 2) how to prevent accumulation of gas in gas pockets in the bowel; and 3) how to eliminate gas from the bowel at the right time in the right way.

Chronic indolent problems of the gut are pervasive. We label them irritable bowel syndrome, spastic colitis, collagenous colitis, ulcerative colitis, Crohn's colitis, diverticulitis, hyper-motility syndrome, leaky gut syndrome, auto-brewery syndrome, the so-called yeast syndrome, intestinal dysbiosis and others. Intractable abdominal bloating is a symptom common to these disorders. I consider these problems essentially disorders of the internal ecology of the bowel. The relevant issues are food incompatibilities, yeast allergy and overgrowth, acid-alkali imbalance, altered bowel flora, parasitic infestation, poor perfusion (insufficient blood flow to the bowel), abnormal bowel motility with episodes of diarrhea, prolonged transit time with constipation, and the resulting disorders of digestion and absorption.

I discuss this subject at length in my monograph *The Altered States of Bowel Ecology and Health Preservation.* The core point of this discussion is this: All these factors impact upon each other and require a holistic, integrated approach to address all the relevant issues. Simple-minded attempts to choose a diagnostic label and prescribe some drug, nutrient or herb do not yield long-term results. Limbic lengthening of back and abdominal muscles followed by ghoraa run *first thing in the morning* offer the best solution to the problem of excessive gas pockets, bloating and cramps. During the ghoraa run, try the following steps:

1.   Sit comfortably and upright in a chair with eyes closed.
2.   Softly repeat the words, "I can sense the space in my abdomen," five times.
3.   "Feel" the space in your abdomen as you gently breathe in and out.
4.   Perceive how the space in your abdomen responds as you breathe in and out.
5.   Softly repeat the words, "I feel the space in my abdomen open up as I breathe in and come together as I breathe out," five times.
6.   Alternate steps # 2 and # 4 for a few minutes until the abdominal space begins to respond.

In ghoraa run, the abdominal muscles gently *message* the loops of bowel — normalizing the normal peristaltic activity of the bowel musculature and speeding up the transit time of the bowel contents. Both factors facilitate the expulsion of the gas during the bowel movement that follows.

ASTHMA AND RESPIRATORY DISORDERS

For respiratory disorders, I recommend ghoraa run and methods of directed pulses and limbic dimension.

We have all heard about exercise-induced asthma and wheezing triggered by cold air. Many of us have also heard of Nancy Hogshead, who suffered from asthma and went on to win the most medals by a swimmer in the 1984 Olympics. Most people have also seen persons with respiratory ailments cough and choke and huff and puff when they are suddenly required to make strenuous physical efforts. How does it all happen? Our lung experts have elaborate theories to explain this and talk about highly specialized lung reflexes, CO_2 retention and neurotransmitter problems. My patients who suffer from asthma and other lung disorders have taught me something different: They simply do not develop respiratory symptoms during limbic exercise. This should not surprise us because the essence of limbic exercise is to be guided by the tissues. In asthma, the bronchial tubes resent sudden exposure to cold air and oxidative stress, and protest by causing spasms and wheezing. When we learn to attend to bronchial responses, they send us the danger signals before they finally close up. The case of competition athletes is different. They need to make a considered choice and may choose to accept drug therapy for a competitive edge.

For chronic respiratory problems including asthma, I recommend methods of limbic dimension, directed pulses and limbic breathing during limbic cycling or ghoraa run. If episodes of wheezing intensifies into an asthma attack, it is preferable to stay with limbic dimensions of the throat or abdomen rather than those of the lungs. Here are simple steps for limbic dimension for lung disorders:

1. Sit comfortably and upright in a chair with eyes closed.
2. Softly repeat the words, "I can imagine the space in my chest cavity," five times.
3. "Feel" the space in the chest cavity as you gently breathe in and out five times.
4. Perceive your chest respond as you breathe in and out.
5. Softly repeat five times the words, "I feel the space in my chest open up as I breathe in and come back together as I breathe out."

6.   Alternate steps #2 and 5 for a few minutes until the chest begins
      to respond.

EXERCISE FOR THE TROUBLED TRIO

The thyroid, pancreas and adrenal glands are a troubled trio of endocrine organs. These organs often bear the brunt of the ever-increasing oxidant stress on human biology. Clinical syndromes caused by oxidant injury to these organs are becoming epidemic in proportion. Recent studies show that thyroid de-iodinase enzymes become impaired and fail to convert inactive precursors to metabolically active thyroid hormones. (It is my strong sense that such enzyme damage will be shown to be oxidative in nature with further research.) Thyroid dysfunction so produced causes problems of low energy and the syndrome of body temperature dysregulation with cold hands and cold feet as the common presenting symptoms. Injury to the pancreas causes syndromes of sugar, insulin and adrenaline roller coasters with symptoms of weakness, mood swings, headache, lightheadedness, sweating and heart palpitations. I discuss this subject at some length in *The Butterfly and Life Span Nutrition*. Injury to the adrenal glands causes the syndrome of chronic stress and suppressed immune and molecular defenses.

Proper management of symptom-complexes that arise from the woes of the troubled trio consists of a holistic, integrated treatment plan. Such a plan should address all elements that increase oxidative stress on human biology and interfere with optimal functions of these organs, including food incompatibility, mold allergy, environmental pollutants, self-regulation, nutrient and herbal therapies, and physical exercise.

HYPOTHYROIDISM AND COLD HANDS AND FEET

For problems of cold hands and feet, I recommend directed pulses, ghoraa run and avoidance of strenuous exercise.

Thyroid hormones are essential for the proper functioning of energy enzymes. Optimal enzyme function, I discuss earlier in this volume, cannot be achieved without slow, sustained exercise. I recommend the method of directed pulses for the problems of body temperature dysregulation for a specific reason: Spasm of arteries is common in hypothyroidism, and autoregulation goes a long way in loosening the tightened arteries and relieving vasospasm in the skin and other body organs.

I know of many people who try to solve the problem of cold hands and feet with programs of strenuous exercise. Such attempts always lead to dismal failures. It is true that strenuous exercise does raise the body temperature for short periods of time due to increased metabolic activity. However, strenuous exercise causes hyperventilation and sweating; both factors promptly cool the body down and undo any benefit that such exercise might bring.

TROUBLESOME HYPERGLYCEMIA-HYPOGLYCEMIC SHIFTS

For troublesome, sharp hyperglycemic-hypoglycemic shifts, I recommend ghoraa run and limbic cycling.

SAD (standard American diet) is in a sad state of affairs. Sugar is the most important anti-nutrient in SAD, and its overload causes dysregulation of sugar-burning enzymes. Human metabolism utilizes three energy sources: carbohydrates, proteins and fats. Historically, the management of hypoglycemia has been based on use of proteins instead of carbohydrates. This approach is usually effective in most instances. For individuals who do not obtain relief of symptoms with this approach, I recommend emphasis on fats as the source of energy and an increase in the daily intake of life span fats. Life span fats in food are the best source of energy. In cases of severe, persistent symptoms caused by sugar-insulin-adrenaline roller coasters, the common advice of increasing proteins in food does not always give the best results — increasing the amount of unoxidized, un-denatured natural life span fats does. Slow, sustained physical activity is as essential for *normalizing* the function of sugar-burning enzymes as it is for up-regulation of fat-burning enzymes. Ghoraa run and limbic cycling are the best exercises for regulating these enzymes.

We have two specific objectives in the management of troublesome hyperglycemic-hypoglycemic shifts that are always followed by insulin and adrenaline roller coasters: 1) normalization of sugar-burning enzymes; and 2) up-regulation of fat-burning enzymes. Both objectives can be achieved by prolonged periods of ghoraa run. I discussed the nutritional therapy for this disorder in *The Butterfly and Life Span Nutrition.* I want to make an essential point here:

LIMBIC EXERCISE FOR CHRONIC ADRENAL STRESS

For the person who suffers from unrelenting stress, I suggest three things: 1) Reach out unto the rising sun; 2) Reach out unto the rising sun; 3) Reach out unto the rising sun.

I have known many people who tried to fight off stress by herculean efforts with strenuous exercise. The benefits of such an approach are limited and temporary. I suggest slow and sustained ghoraa run or limbic cycling. Persons who suffer from severe stress should prepare themselves for the bites of the limbic dog before the full benefits of limbic exercise become apparent to them. Now I return to the rising sun.

The eastern sky has unique healing powers. No affirmations have the carrying capacity of the deep clear of the morning sky. No sight can be as comforting as the clouds underlit by the rising sun. No words of wisdom can be as enlightening as the limbic language of silence. In unrelenting stress, the limbic dog bites relentlessly. When the anguished tissues rebel, the energy of life becomes difficult to perceive.

The fingertips refuse to pulse. The arms stay limp. The muscles in the torso turn and twist. The bowel bloats, and the heart races and flutters. Sparks fly under the skin. The distortions of the mind become insufferable. The chemistry of the tissues becomes that of fireworks on the fourth of July. Tranquilizers stop working. The psychiatrist's words ring hollow. The preacher's exhortations seem distant. When all else fails, the rising sun and the eastern sky offers a reprieve. The language of silence provides a link with that larger *presence* that always surrounds us.

Frivolous notions of a delusional idealogue! Some people might muse at my words.

LIMBIC EXERCISE FOR THE ELDERLY

For the elderly, no issue is more critical in physical fitness than the issue of limbic lengthening.

When tissues age, their metabolic requirements and needs for physical activity change. Still it does not justify the common practice of blaming age for common maladies.

I have been told exercise improves the cognitive functions of the aged. I do not know much about the cognitive functions of the aged — or for that matter of the young — and so I cannot say whether exercise does or does not improve it. I do know exercise makes elderly people feel better physically, and that whatever makes people feel better physically must lift their spirits and improve their mental and emotional status. They can think clearly because their minds are not fogged out with stagnant enzyme systems. With advancing age, muscle fibers lose protein and shrink, ligaments and connective tissue accumulate stiff — oxidized and denatured — scleroprotein molecules and lose elasticity, bones lose matrix and minerals and thin out. All these elements lead to loss of fluidity and resilience in the connective tissue, muscles and bone. Limbic lengthening of the connective tissue prepares the tissues for freer motion. Slow and sustained exercise prevents loss of length and strength of muscle fibers and promotes new bone formation. I might add here that there is a loss of fluidity of motion of the connective tissue and muscles that comes with passing years, not just for the elderly but for everyone.

USE IT OR LOSE IT

This may be an overutilized phrase, but it does carry a nugget of truth. There is an essential message here for the elderly. Life is living — and living for the connective tissue and muscles is motion. Physical inactivity is a punishment for the aging tissues. So it is for each muscle fascicle, each ligament band and each tendon sheath and fiber. *Disabling* musculoskeletal restrictions often arrive with arthritis, tendinitis, bursitis, myositis, fibromyalgia and related disorders to which the elderly are especially prone. Many commonly used exercises are too strenuous for the injured tissues and increase the inflammatory response in such conditions.

There are many forms of hydrotherapy that are appropriate for the elderly with connective tissue and muscle difficulties. These exercises can be learned from the area physiotherapists, and special arrangements can be made to do them frequently with eyes closed and without competitive goals at home.

LIMBIC EXERCISE FOR CHRONIC FATIGUE

For chronic fatigue, I recommend limbic cycling in the initial stages and ghoraa run in later stages after the energy level significantly improves with nondrug therapies. The key element is not to force any additional stress on exhausted tissues.

Jackie, a 38-year-old woman, consulted me for incapacitating chronic fatigue. As a teenager, she was very athletic. She was quite health-conscious and had maintained an active exercise schedule even after she had three children. She had been given prolonged tetracycline therapy for acne and had received multiple courses of antibiotic therapy for recurrent episodes of sore throat and bronchitis that were in reality allergic symptoms. She knew she was allergic, but her allergies had never been diagnosed and managed properly with desensitization.

In tears, Jackie told me of her struggle to pull herself out of her debilitating fatigue with heroic efforts to exercise even when it caused severe pain.

"I work hard at it. I push myself even though I feel my muscles are being torn apart. Sometimes I think it helps a little, but then I collapse again," she said.

Some people who do research in the so-called chronic fatigue syndrome amuse me. They harness their exhausted patients with sore limbs and aching muscles into their computerized ergometric machines. Next, they demand from their injured and energy-depleted tissues to perform according to what *they* — the researchers — think is best for these patients. The researchers then conclude that exercise causes spasms of the blood vessels in the limbic system of their brains and leads to vasoconstriction and inadequate blood supply. Should this really surprise us? Why wouldn't these frightened blood vessels tighten up when molested by the clever designs of these brilliant researchers?

People who suffer from chronic disabling fatigue do need exercise, but not of the type that our "researchers" teach us. They do not need exercise that further injures hurt muscles. Exercises for patients with chronic fatigue must be slow, sustained and nontraumatic. In other words, it must be limbic. It frequently requires patient and persistent efforts to improve physical stamina. An excellent way to build stamina is to do limbic exercises for brief periods of a few minutes several times during the day.

I discuss the subject of chronic fatigue at length in *The Canary and Chronic Fatigue*. For a discussion of the biochemical and energetic basis of chronic fatigue, I refer the professional reader to my article *Chronic Fatigue Is a State of Accelerated Oxidative Molecular Damage* published in the 1993 syllabus of the American Academy of Environmental Medicine, Denver.

Chronic fatigue is an energy dysfunction — a state of failure of the enzymes that are involved with the process of energy generation. The roles played by viruses, Epstein-Barr and others, in the causation of chronic fatigue are secondary in nature. I have cared for a large number of people with debilitating chronic fatigue. Almost all such patients have demonstrable mold and/or food allergy, have been given multiple courses of antibiotics and have clinical and laboratory evidence of impaired immune status *before* they develop chronic fatigue.

Here, I want to make three essential points about disabling chronic fatigue. First, chronic fatigue is a *reversible* disorder for almost all patients except those with paralyzing chemical sensitivity. Second, it cannot be reversed with drugs. Drugs, especially the toxic antiviral drugs, do sometimes give temporary relief, but the patient pays dearly for such short-term relief. Third, optimal management of chronic fatigue requires full and equal emphasis on all the following areas: 1) recognition and nondrug management of food and mold allergy; 2) use of carefully formulated oral and intravenous nutrient protocols; 3) diagnosis and removal of toxic metal load; 4) autoregulation for turning the turbulent energy dynamics of fatigue — a tissue chemistry of the fireworks of the fourth of July — into the even and sustained energy dynamics of health; 5) limbic exercise; 6) strict avoidance of antibiotics except for truly life threatening infections; and 7) strict avoidance of insecticides, fungicides and other toxic molecules.

LIMBIC EXERCISE FOR OBESITY

For obesity, I recommend the following: 1) Do not —repeat do not —join a weight loss program that serves up toxic, packaged frozen foods; 2) Learn well the differences between foods that support fat-burning enzymes and those that injure them; 3) Begin a steady program of slow and sustained limbic exercises; and 4) Prepare for coping with the bites of the limbic dog, perhaps for long periods of time.

Does obesity ever reach a stage of irreversibility? If it does, how can anyone recognize this? These are some of the most vexing questions I have faced when caring for grossly obese people.

Whenever I encourage my grossly obese patients — men and women 120, 150 or more pounds overweight — my thoughts wander around and then settle on two questions: 1) Do fat cells ever become gangrenous just as the feet and legs? 2) If the fat cells are really mortuaries of dead fat molecules, what's the point of any weight loss program?

Dead enzymes, evidently, cannot be up-regulated. Just as we accept the necessity of amputating a gangrenous leg to save the life, do we need to amputate dead fat cells? These thoughts are depressing for me. I do not write about dead and dying fat cells to offer license to our plastic surgery community to expand their assault on body fat anymore than they already have. The very notion of correcting serious catabolic maladaptation with surgical scalpels is offensive to me.

I write about dead and dying fat cells so that severely obese people may understand the true depth of their problems. They need to brace themselves for the many and prolonged bites of the limbic dog. In the chapter, The Cortical Monkey and Limbic Dog, I relate the stories of Edward and Sheila for specific reasons. The problem of severe obesity can be just as indolent and cause just as much anguish as deep, unremitting depression or severe autoimmune disorders. Overweight people need to understand that the limbic dog bites not because it is vengeful and seeks revenge but because the joys of kindness and love are alien to him. There may be as many as 100 trillion cells in the human body. Except for nerve and some muscle cells, these cells die and are replaced with new cells at all times. The process of fat cells dying and being replaced with new fat cells may become very slow in the grossly obese person, but it doesn't stop altogether. Obese people must know this no matter how sharp or hard or unremitting the bites of the limbic dog become.

Whenever I hear of exercise prescriptions for severely obese people, I cannot help but think of the torture that exercise is for them. Walking, jogging or cycling for losing excess pounds of body fat are punishing propositions, illusions of slimness that inevitably will be torn apart by the ugly reality of aching muscles, sore ligaments and bruised spirits. Minutes of exercise turn into hours of sheer misery for them. I wonder how their fat-burning enzymes will respond to the persistent demands of their thinking heads. I wonder how the cortical monkey will pour heavy loads of oxidizing stress molecules onto their sluggish enzymes. What are their chances against such odds? How long will they persist? How much can they endure?

The punishment seems to last forever. The illusions of burning fat with exercise and melting fat with special diets endure. The fat cells stay bloated. The muscles continue to hurt. The fat seems to solidify, even more densely. How do these people turn the punishment of exercise into periods of deep, visceral silence? How do they banish their cortical monkeys? How will the limbic dogs cease to bite?

I know what obese people need — time for a deeper renewal, not only of the tissues burdened with fat overload, but of their entire *being*. This, of course, is easier said than done for many obese people with bloated fat cells, impoverished enzymes and past hurts of broken promises of weight loss. The sharp bites of the limbic dog are the only true experiences they have had in their battle of pounds. Their bloated cells resent the demands put upon them by our weight control experts — and by their slick and cruel commercials that promise them the lithesome bodies of some models in beach scenes. They struggle, sweat and curse to lose weight, and then go on to regain whatever pounds they lost — and some more. The paralyzed enzymes stay paralyzed, the bloated cells continue to bloat. The tissues do respond — finally when we learn to listen to them. Also, the tissues do have a gentle guiding energy that leads us out of our cortical tunnels into the limbic openness. This is the essence of autoregulation. Overweight people need to *know* all this.

The ancients understood two things about human metabolism: 1) It can be slowed down by fasting or eating less; and 2) It can be it speeded up by *eating more* and by *doing more physical activity*. The third element they didn't seem to have predicted is that toxic chemicals can poison metabolic enzymes and cause obesity. I discuss at length the enzyme derangements and the food choices that cause obesity in the chapters, On the Nature of Obesity and The Catabolic Maladaptation in *The Butterfly and Life Span Nutrition*. I strongly urge the overweight reader to read and reread these chapters.

There are four groups of risk factors that lead to obesity: nutritional factors, environmental factors, stress and lack of physical fitness. All successful strategies for achieving the optimal life span weight must address all four groups of risk factors. *Dieting doesn't work.* Food fuels the furnace of human metabolism; exercise stokes its fires. The only way excess fat can be lost is by up-regulating fat-burning enzymes. And the only way fat-burning enzymes can be up-regulated is by eating more and doing more slow, sustained exercise. Specifically, the best type of exercise for achieving and maintaining life span weight loss, in my judgment, is ghoraa run. Limbic cycling with an exercise cycle is my next best choice for those who are unable to do ghoraa run due to some health disorder.

MYOFASCIAL TRIGGER POINTS AND MEMBRANE POTENTIAL DERANGEMENTS

I include some brief comments in this chapter about the diagnosis and treatment of myofascial trigger points and cell membrane potential derangements for two practical reasons: 1) These painful disorders are the principal physical reasons why many people are forced to relinquish their exercise programs; and 2) These disorders, with rare exceptions, can usually be treated with safe, nondrug therapies. Injection into these points of 50% glucose solution with 2% xylocaine anesthetic solution evokes a powerful proliferative healing response, the so-called prolotherapy. Neural therapy with injection of 1% xylocaine into areas of scar formation and chronic pain are often very successful for relief of pain.

Myofascial trigger points are tender, painful areas located within tendons, ligaments and other types of connective tissue. Less commonly, these points are located within the bodies of muscles, probably at neuromuscular junctions. These trigger points develop when the connective tissue fibers, and less commonly, muscle fibers, are torn or ruptured by injury. Most such injuries heal spontaneously with rest, and do not lead to formation of chronic painful trigger points. If the natural process of healing is impaired or arrested by ongoing mechanical stresses on the injured areas, the torn or ruptured fibers do not heal and a myofascial trigger point forms. Injured myofascial fibers get wound up so tightly that spontaneous un-winding becomes unlikely.

The membrane potential derangements are ill-understood disorders of chronic pain. Such points are thought to be caused by certain energy events that interfere with changes that occur in normal nerve cell membrane potentials.

Two diagrams that follow show the structure of ligaments that stabilize the ankle joint in health and irregular tears and lacerations in the same ligaments that lead to the formation of painful trigger points.

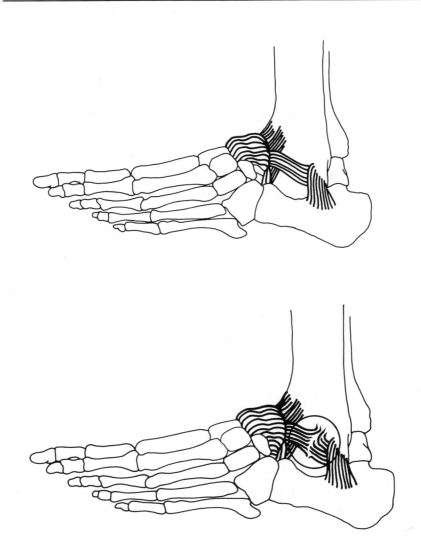

The purpose of the injection of one-half to one ml of 50% glucose injection into the area of torn ligament is to stimulate the proliferative repair response of the injured tissues. This is the reason such therapy is called proliferative therapy or prolotherapy. Many other types of solutions to stimulate the healing response of torn tissues have been used. My preference for 50% glucose solution with equal amounts of 2% xylocaine as anesthetic is based on positive clinical results I have observed with this material. Diagnosis and successful treatment of myofascial trigger points and scars with prolotherapy and/or neural therapy require considerable skill and experience on the part of the physician. The search for such an individual may be time-consuming but is well worth the effort because the results in terms of relief of pain are far superior than those obtained with drugs. Many members of the American College for Advancement in Medicine are experienced with techniques of prolotherapy and neural therapies (714-583-7666). Of course, when performed by knowledgeable professionals, there are no serious side effects of such therapies.

****

In close this chapter and end this book by returning to the central ideas with which I started: Health is not possible without optimal efficiency of energy enzymes, and that energy enzymes poisoned by oxidized, denatured foods and physical inactivity cannot be up-regulated by dieting or by exercise programs to "burn" fat. Physical exercise is more giving when we allow the tissues to lead us; the mind cannot molest the injured tissues for too long. We cannot clever-think our way out of all our problems. Exercise for the whole life span requires the limbic language of silence.

Success in autoregulation and in limbic exercises calls for preparedness. Preparedness for communicating with the language of silence and for perceiving the tissue energy. Preparedness for banishing the cortical clutter. Preparedness for receiving, and not for demanding. Preparedness for gratitude, and not for greed. Preparedness for limbic images if any should take form in the limbic openness spread wide before us. Preparedness for perceiving the energy of living tissues and for allowing ourselves to be guided this gentle energy. Preparedness for living within the moment. Preparedness for higher states of consciousness. Preparedness for spirituality, that essential link between man and that larger *presence* that surrounds him at all times.

Throughout history, the most common debilitating human ailment has been cold feet.

Unknown

Index

In praise of Majid Ali's *The Cortical Monkey and Healing*

" .... people who read this book will benefit from it." Linus Pauling

"If anyone else told me of Majid Ali's dictum, I would disbelieve it all. Majid's expertise in so many fields makes disregarding anything he says a costly mistake. He has taught me autoregulation, and I have personally seen what it alone can do."

Hueston King, M.D., Past President
American Academy of Otolaryngic Allergy

"This is a fascinating book coming from a physician who was a surgeon who became a pathologist, immunologist, allergist, ecologist, and now a teacher in self-regulation. There are many little gems here."

Norman Shealy, M.D., Past President
American Holistic Medical Association

"The new book ... is a wonderful overview of the problems with standard medical care. Dr. Ali mixes fact with philosophy into a unique and readable book. One can now clearly understand the illogic of modern medicine and the logic of molecular medicine."

James Frackleton, M.D., Past President
American College for Advancement in Medicine

"It contains many fresh insights and much common sense. I intend to use it as a primary reference during my medical students teaching sessions this fall."

Jessica Davis, M.D.
Cornell Medical Center, New York

In praise of Majid Ali's *The Butterfly and Life Span Nutrition*

"I believe the wisdom it contains can profoundly affect the health of our people and the health policy of our nation and the world."

Michael Schachter, M.D., Past President
American College for Advancement in Medicine

" ... is a masterly blend of the intuitive wisdom of the ancients with the basic chemistry of life. The result is an enormously valuable book for those interested in nutrition and fitness."

Hueston King, M.D., Past President
American Academy of Otolaryngic Allergy

"If you are going to read but one book about your health this year, please make it *The Butterfly and Life Span Nutrition.*"

Francis Waickman, M.D., Past President
American Academy of Environmental Medicine

"If there were only a way to ensure that every medical student and resident had access to this material, it would be a great boon to the health of mankind. For ourselves we will be honored to have, to show, to learn, to teach and to practice from these texts."

Jerrold Finnie, M.D. and Dolores Finnie, R.N., New York